FOUNTAIN OF YOUTH
EXERCISES

FOR VITALITY, RADIANCE, JOY & FULFILLMENT IN

FIFTEEN MINUTES

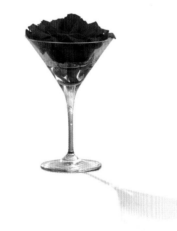

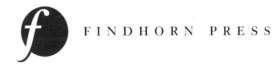

FINDHORN PRESS

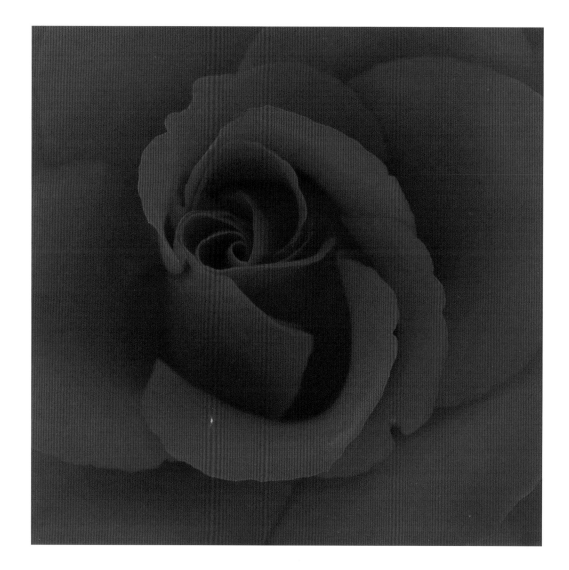

If I were to wish for anything,
I should not wish for wealth and power,
but for the passionate sense of the potential,
for the eye which, ever young and ardent,
sees the possible…
what wine is so sparkling, so fragrant, so intoxicating,
as possibility!

~ SOREN KIERKEGAARD

Fountain of Youth Exercises

for Vitality, Radiance, Joy & Fulfillment in

Fifteen Minutes

A RECIPE FOR LONGEVITY BY

Naomi Sophia Call

 FINDHORN PRESS

ISBN 978-1-84409–528–5

The exercises in this book are safe and gentle. If you have unmedicated
high blood pressure, eye inflamations or any reason to question
the suitability of the exercises, please consult with your doctor first.
The publisher and author disclaim all liability in connection with the
use of the information in individual cases.

British Library Cataloguing-in-Publication Data.
A Catalogue record for this book is available from the British Library

Cover, interior design by Damian Keenan
Cover & interior photographs by Naomi Sophia Call
Five Rite photographers Auston Call & Donna Jacobsen
Author photographs by Loghan Call & Ian Robson
Back cover author photograph by Auston Call
Printed and bound in the European Union

1 2 3 4 5 6 7 8 9 10 16 15 14 13 12 11

Published by
Findhorn Press
117-121 High Street,
Forres IV36 1AB,
Scotland, UK

t +44 (0)1309 690582
f +44 (0)131 777 2711
e info@findhornpress.com
www.findhornpress.com

the ingredients

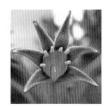
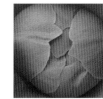
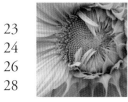
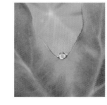

the ingredients

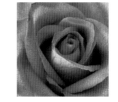
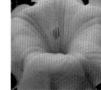
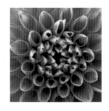

the ingredients

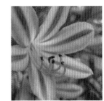
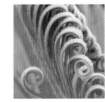
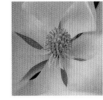
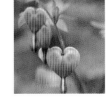

For my mother Mary Jane…

and your forever youthful passions

for my father Jack…

building countless best moments

and to all of my ancestors

~ Thank you

thank you... thank you...

Words fall short of the depth of my gratitude. I cherish the blessing that you all are to me, to this book and to our world.

Thierry Bogliolo and Findhorn Press for your choice, trust and patience to share my ideas with the world. For all of the times you stretched with me to bring this vision to its fullness, I am deeply grateful. Findhorn Gardens for opening and affirming to the world, the inherent magic that abounds on our Earth.

Deborah Doyle for your literary brilliance, friendship and wisdom. Gerri Merrielle, from the first murmur of conception you were there again. Taylor Call for your wealth of information and support through editing, and life. Donna Jacobsen for your loving support in countless ways, not to mention your t-shirt.

Megan Pincus Katijani for serendipitously becoming my editor... your extraordinary labor support and fortuitous pearls of wisdom are the the icing on the cake. Thank you for perfecting the recipe!

Damian Keenan, for your graphic perfection, patience and perseverance throughout a spiritual journey across an ocean and thousands of miles enabling us to co-create this work of art, and be blessed to get to know one another.

Gail Torr for being there with your shining light, and helping me to shine mine.

Auston Call & Donna Jacobsen for photographing my mother and I in The Five Rites. Loghan Call & Ian Robson for photos of me.

the models

Models are volunteer students who were photographed on chilly winter mornings in southern California. Their love of yoga and pre-dawn sense of adventure is a gift and inspiration to us all. A special thank you to Bill, Carolyn, Helen and Ian whose photos were unfortunately not used, your spirit is equally appreciated. Also a big thank you to Gary.

Patty Arambarri, *65 years young*
Julia Burgess-Perrot, *74 years young*
Mary Jane Call, *79 youthful years*
Brigit Clark-Smith, *82 years young*
Marla Daigh, *56 years young*
Vic Freudenberger, *91 years young*
Mary Hansom, *69 years young*
Donna Jacobsen, *65 years young*
Jan O'Hara, *60 youthful years*
Heather Martin, *57 years young*
Tony Matarrese, *57 youthful years*
Pat Miller, *77 years young*
Cap Strawser, *89 years young*
Harry Tracy, *57 years young*

To my family and friends, your loving, inspiring support in countless ways, between every word… is the leavening in my life.

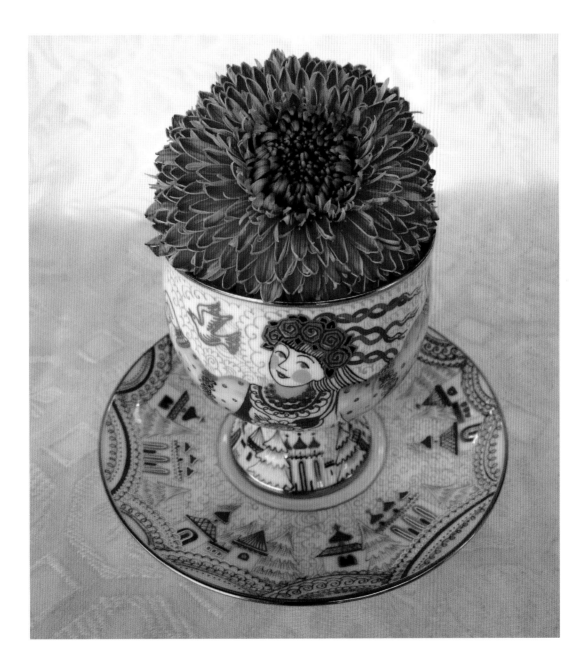

Living is the art of loving.
Sharing is the art of living.

~ *BOOKER T. WASHINGTON*

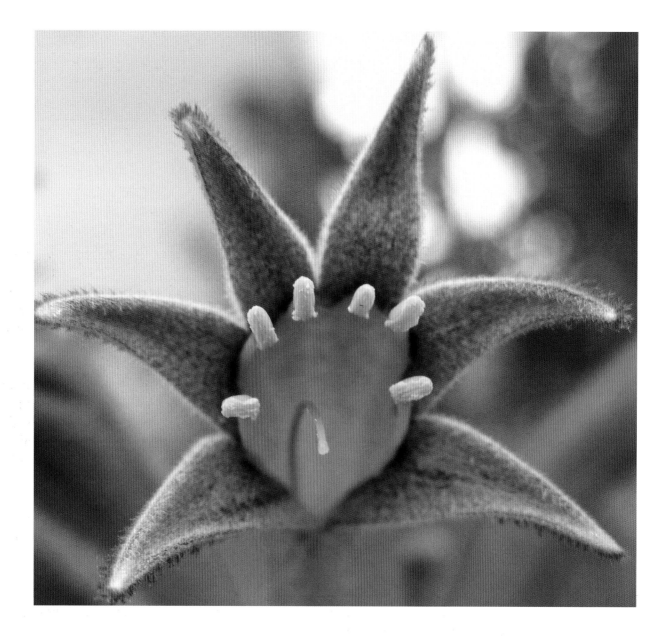

To find joy in work
is to discover
the fountain of youth.

~ PEARL S. BUCK

"Paying it Forward"

As I reflect on my life's journey, the people who have enriched my life and my desire to make a difference in the world, I am present to the concept of "pay it forward." This is the title of a movie from 2000, about a boy who comes up with the idea to pay good deeds forward, rather than back, and in turn, transforms the lives of an ever-widening circle of people. I believe, as a teacher, life coach, chef and healer, in "paying forward" the gifts that I have been given on this path to health, radiance, happiness and longevity.

My journey began in the 1970's, when I learned of macrobiotics from my sister Kimberly. I had recently become a vegetarian and was transitioning from a standard American diet. My revelations led me to studies pioneered by Michio and Aveline Kushi, who brought an inspired vision, a tantalizingly beautiful cuisine and a refreshing way of life to my family. I am grateful to my teachers and especially the Kushi's, whose profound philosophy has continued on and inspired millions of people around the world. *(www.kushiinstitute.org)*

As my studies deepened, my mother introduced me to The Five Rites, often referred to as "the secret to the fountain of youth." Peter Kelder brought these exercises to the general public in his 1930's book entitled, *The Ancient Secret to the Fountain of Youth*.

Years later, my sister Taylor met Dr. Tienko Ting, who is originally from Taiwan and currently resides in the United States. Ting discovered what he calls Natural Chi Movement (*www.naturalchimovement.com*). I thank them both for adding this significant ingredient to my practice and teaching.

Many of the yoga stretches woven into this book are central to my work at retirement communities. It is an unequalled inspiration to witness the courage and desire of students practicing, and often beginning, yoga in their 70's, 80's and 90's. The beauty of yoga is that it can be easily modified for any body. I have no doubt that regular, conscious exercise can absolutely contribute to a longer and healthier life. I thank my elder students for further crystallizing this faith that was introduced to me by my Kripalu yoga teachers. *(www.kripalu.org)*

For almost 20 years, Michael Shaffer, my chiropractor, friend and intuitive healer, has illuminated my path and helped me to see who I truly am. I feel divinely blessed.

The flower photos interspersed throughout this book represent a tiny glimpse of a favorite teacher… nature. The miracle and beauty of nature brings me into my heart and spirit over and over. Flowers to me are heaven on Earth. Their endless array of colors, shapes and intoxicating aromas will forever inspire me. All of life is a gift.

I am deeply grateful for all of these Beings over the last 30 years, and to be given the opportunities to share my blessings with thousands of people, and now, with you. In the spirit of paying it forward, and casting our pearls, I hope that you too may become inspired to be a link in the lineage of this ancient, re-discovered and newly connected wisdom.

To all of my teachers… including all of my students, for you are my teachers and mirrors, radiantly reflecting and inspiring me to grow and expand every day of my life… I offer my eternal gratitude.

Namaste.

This is your life.
It is your time as you…
experience everything good

– MAYA ANGELOU

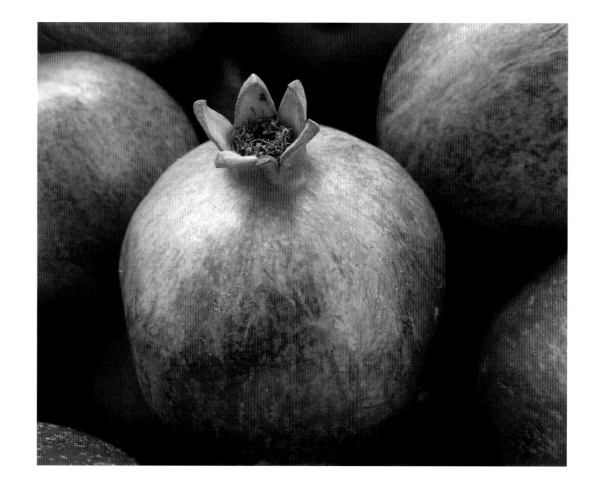

When I walk into my kitchen today, I am not alone.
Whether we know it or not, none of us is.
We bring fathers and mothers and kitchen tables,
and every meal we have ever eaten.
Food is never just food.
It's a way of getting at something else:
who we are, who we have been,
and who we want to be.

~ MOLLY WIZENBERG

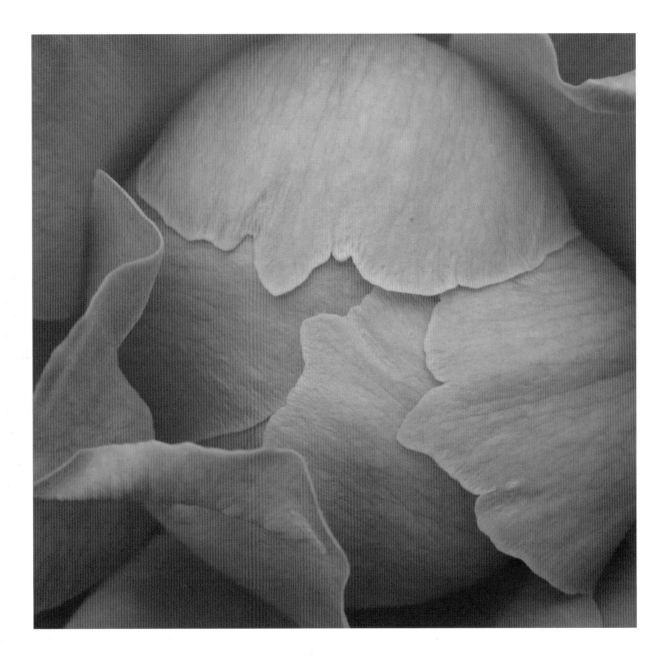

Youth has no age.

~ PABLO PICASSO

Introduction:
a recipe for longevity

During my three decades as a healing arts professional, scores of students of all ages — a great many, like the models in this book, who are over age 55 — have told me that I have given them fresh inspiration, renewed energy and eliminated countless symptoms and complaints. What I teach them about youthfulness cannot easily be encapsulated under one heading, as my work encompasses an array of exercises and tips gathered not only from my experience in the field of natural health, but also from our ancestors centuries ago.

Because this can sound overwhelming to a person trying to juggle the demands of life, I prefer to simplify these youth-enhancing exercises into small segments — just fifteen minutes at a time — that can be incorporated into anyone's daily life. Given my background as a chef, I like to envision this as a "recipe for longevity." Just as we prepare a holiday feast — following each small step then allowing our dishes to simmer or bake as we move onto something else — we can use this recipe, in fifteen-minute steps at a time, to prepare our bodies, minds and spirits for a long and vibrant life.

The Recipe in Practice

My "recipe for longevity" includes exercises and tips that can refresh, strengthen and beautify the body, focus the mind, and blossom the spirit. These exercises are commonly referred to as practices, as they are usually performed on a daily basis. We have learned that consistency makes a measurable difference in our overall results. A little exercise each day usually results in our feeling better than if we did it all in one day a week. Every society around the globe known for longevity shares the common component of daily exercise.

The exercises in this book are ancient, revered practices that have evolved over thousands of years throughout a number of countries. The primary practices presented in Fountain of Youth Exercises – the core ingredients of my "recipe for longevity" -- are: Conscious Breathing, Do-In, The Five Rites, Yoga, and Meditation in Motion. I also add to the practice the important ingredients of healthy diet, mental exercise, and practicing gratitude, to round out the care and feeding of our bodies, minds, and spirits. When masterfully mixed together — one small step at a time — I have seen time and again how these ingredients lead people of any age to sustained, youthful vitality, clarity and happiness. Isn't this what we all imagine we could find at the *Fountain of Youth*?

Overview of Ingredients

Breathing is something we don't have to think about, though it deserves our attention. Conscious breathing can help improve the functioning of our bodies, balance our emotions, clear our minds, and increase our longevity. As our respiratory rate slows down, every system in our body responds in kind.

Do-In (dough - een) is an ancient revered practice of stimulating one's energy or *chi* (chee), through a series of movements. This energy is also known as *ki* in Japan, *prana* in India and Tibet, *wakan* by the Lakotas, *orenda* by the Iroquois and *Holy Spirit* in Christian tradition, to name a few. Do-In is also used as a daily preventive measure and self-diagnostic tool. Long regarded as precious secrets, Do-In techniques were verbally passed on through family generations.

The Five Rites, commonly referred to as "The Ancient Secret to The Fountain of Youth," are exercises that were created and performed by Tibetan monks and first brought to the United States in the 1930's. The Rites energize and strengthen every major muscle group, meridian, organ, chakra and system in the body.

Yoga is a practice that has gained enormous popularity during the past ten years. Earlier, it too was only known to isolated groups and held in an esteemed and sacred fashion. Fifteen minutes of poses that I feel are especially beneficial, doable, and complement the Five Rites are highlighted. I encourage you, over time, to develop your own repertoire of choices. If the poses in this book are too strenuous, you may want to refer to *Yoga in Bed: Awaken Body, Mind, and Spirit in Fifteen Minutes (naomicall.com)*.

Life would be infinitely happier if we could only be born at the age of 80 and gradually approach 18.
~ MARK TWAIN, IN HIS TWILIGHT YEARS

Most people know that stress is a leading factor in premature aging. Meditation and Meditation in Motion are key contributors to health and longevity. The modern-day quest to master multi-tasking is being re-evaluated as we come to understand that mindfulness and simplicity, reminiscent of our elders' lifestyle, are the keys to a healthier and more fulfilling life.

Along with these practices, the most important core ingredient in this recipe for longevity is the understanding that the body must be, first and foremost, well nourished, well rested, breathing fresh air and drinking *pure* water. Prioritizing and creating a home, workplace and body that are free from pesticides and chemical contaminants, inside and out, are foundational to longevity. The mind and spirit also need regular "exercise."

It is good to have an end to journey towards, but it is the journey that matters…

~ URSULA LEGUIN

Every day we have countless blessings. Creating time to be present with our blessings and to our cups being not simply half full, but overflowing, opens and strengthens one's heart and spirit. Reverence is like leavening — the ingredient that will elevate our every step and bring us closer to realizing our dreams.

Fifteen-Minute Steps

As you familiarize yourself with these practices, you will be drawn to some more than others, and those preferences may change over time. Trust your intuition; do not force your body. Many people simply cannot find an hour in their day to exercise or care for themselves, though fifteen minutes is findable. Little snippets are often welcome reprieves from the computer or phone, and with focus and intention can deeply revitalize you.

As many times throughout your day as possible, pause and replenish yourself. It is best to accomplish your first goal of fifteen minutes when you awaken. Begin your day with nourishing you, before anyone or anything else. Create fifteen minutes for yourself before lunch, and again when your workday ends as a gentle transition. Moments speckled throughout your day that are focused can be more potent than one session that feels compressed or stressful to fit in.

When we are striving to de-habituate unconscious behaviors, the continuity and repetition of conscious activity throughout our day will eradicate unconscious patterns more efficiently. Taking care of yourself is the most important gift that you can give to your family and to yourself. Prioritizing one's well-being and radiance, internally and externally, quickly leads to more energy and longevity.

One or two days a week you might dedicate to do the Five Rites and yoga, and the alternate days you could diversify with Do-in and Meditation in Motion. Begin and close your practices with focused breathing and mindfulness to enliven every aspect of your life. Find *your* rhythm, trust, and enjoy your self-discovery!

The "Fountain of Youth": A Brief History

Although it is the Spanish explorer Juan Ponce de Leon in the16th-century who is most linked to the search for the Fountain of Youth, there were many others before him. The quest for going "somewhere" to find this self-contained elixir of life has certainly proven elusive.

As far back as 323 B.C., reports note that Alexander the Great had searched for a river alleged to bring youth. In the 12th century A.D., legends tell of a king who ruled a land known for its river of gold and fountain of youth. From Bimini to Ethiopia, there are stories about the "water of life" and unfulfilled quests.

Alchemists throughout time in ancient China, India and the West have dedicated countless years of their lives to creating the elixir, often referred to as the "Quintessence of Life." Scientists today spend millions of dollars in research striving to extend and enhance life as we know it.

To date, the elderly visitors who sip the sulfur-smelling waters at the Fountain of Youth Archeological Park in St. Augustine, Florida, in the United States have not become visibly more youthful. And research in laboratories across the globe has not unearthed the answer to eternal youth. Interestingly, people continue to search outside of themselves for the answer.

Far from laboratories, and long before the written word, indigenous people were dedicating their lives to understanding their bodies in such a way that they were enhancing the longevity of their lives and our lives. Their collected wisdom informs the practices in this book — exercises and movements that have been performed for hundreds, if not thousands, of years.

As we learn what vital indigenous people believed, I feel it is crucial to our well-being that we integrate their inner knowing into our own body, mind and spirit. To truly preserve our youthful energy, we need to feed our bodies with rejuvenating exercises, fresh air and a wholesome diet, our minds with challenges, and our spirits with our passions. The real Fountain of Youth lies within this commitment to our whole selves.

Youth is not a time of life;
it is a state of mind;
it is not a matter of rosy
cheeks, red lips
and supple knees;
it is a matter of the will,
a quality of the
imagination, a vigor of
the emotions;
it is the freshness of the
deep springs of life.
~ SAMUEL ULLMAN

Getting Started

Choose a quiet place where you can focus without distractions. Outdoors in nature is ideal. Proximity to trees or flowers will enhance your experience. Trees have an enormous amount of chi (life force) that enlivens every breath you take. If you practice indoors, opening a window or a door, even a crack, can enhance your well-being.

Once you have learned to focus and deepen your breathing, you can do these exercises anywhere you are comfortable. I even practice Do-In sitting in traffic in my car. The exercises can be done while watching TV or shared with others. Children often enjoy the inherent playfulness of Do-In. As we know, laughter is great medicine!

You may choose to remove your metal jewelry. Some practitioners believe metal interferes with the flow of chi. Experiment to determine what is best for you.

It is important to have an empty bladder and an empty belly, especially when you practice yoga. Choose comfortable, loose-fitting clothing that will not restrict any part of your body. Music is optional, and for some, greatly enhances their meditation-in-motion practice.

Open your mind. The power of our thoughts is fundamental to the well-being of our body, mind and spirit. I encourage you to approach your exercises as though you are doing them for the first time. Allow new possibilities to be effortless by not imposing self-limiting thoughts. Instead, visualize your next goals already being accomplished.

Pause often throughout your practice to experience and acknowledge the difference you are making. Take your time with the exercises, allow your thoughts to focus on the moment. The more mindfulness, the better the result. This may add enlightening or releasing moments to the early stages of your practice that are well worth the added time.

Bring your awareness to your body, mind and spirit, with every breath. Honor your body and your visions of what you believe in *your heart* to be possible. Feel your boundless, youthful joy, and make these minutes count! Be here now.

TIP: If you wear jewelry, particularly silver, you may wish to see if you notice a difference in your energy and circulation by removing your jewelry at night. Wearing silver jewelry can have a "cold" effect on the body. If you tend to already feel cold, or have cold fingers and feet, experiment with wearing jewelry on special occasions instead of daily.

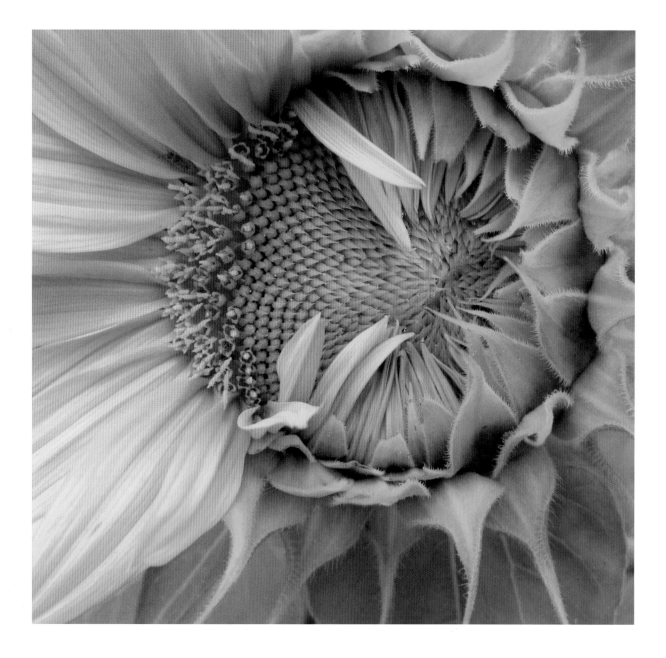

The quieter you become,
the more you can hear.

~ RAM DASS

Conscious Breath:
the elixir of life

Each breath is a new beginning in your body. Breathing is a cornerstone to the quantity of your energy, and the quality of your life. Changing your relationship to your breathing — from unconscious or second-nature to conscious and intentional — can dramatically change your overall health and vitality.

For all of us, our breath is crucial to each moment of our being, and we receive many physical benefits from deep breathing. Some of the most documented are:

— Lowers blood pressure, metabolic rate and blood sugar
— Helps to regulate digestion and elimination
— Aids the detoxification process
— Enables every other system in the body to relax in response
— Improves and increases the amount and delivery of oxygen to the organs
— Eases stress, nervousness and anxiety

When you take in a full, deep breath, your diaphragm is able to move down into your abdominal area, and your lungs can then expand more completely into your chest cavity. This can only happen when your *belly is expanding with your inhalation and retracting with your exhalation.*

The diaphragm is connected to the lower rib cage and ultimately the lumbar area of the spine. A deep breath into the diaphragm naturally massages and detoxifies organs and tissues, enhances circulation and supports the lymphatic system. Every system ultimately benefits from deep breathing, including the function and focus of the brain.

We also know that hormones and emotions are stabilized with regular deep breathing. People who practice breathing exercises tend to have less illness as the immune system also becomes stronger. We simply feel better and happier. When we breathe more consciously, we have more energy. This breath awareness and application is an important key to longevity.

Breathing as an Exercise

- Begin by finding a comfortable and quiet place to sit, preferably outside. Position yourself as upright as possible because posture is vital to acquiring a deep breath.

You may want to experiment with placing a cushion underneath the tip of your tailbone. This can enable your pelvis to shift forward, and your spine to become more upright.

We tend to breathe "backwards" to what is natural, with a contracting motion on inhaling. But if you observe something filling with air, it expands. Imagine a yellow balloon for example. See the balloon expanding. Now close your eyes and imagine your belly is that balloon. This may feel *very* unnatural at first!

- Placing your palm over your navel can help you to focus and bring a deeper connection. As you breathe in, press your abdominal muscle out into your palm.
- As you exhale, apply a gentle pressure with your hand to help expel the air. Use this gentle assistance for as long as you find it helpful. Practice this breath for a few minutes.

If you feel light headed, simply return to your normal breathing and the dizziness will subside. If practicing during the day, face toward the sun. Align your intention to draw in this positive energy and new beginning, enlivening every cell in your body.

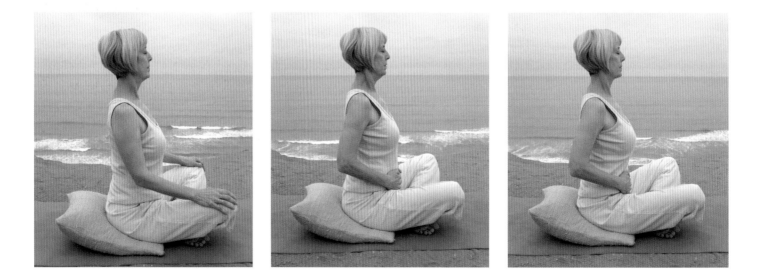

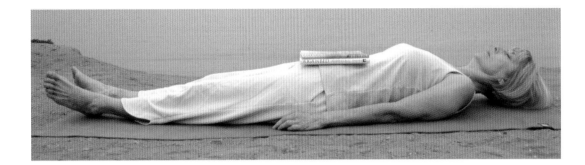

It is a joy to sit,
stable and at ease,
and return to
our breathing,
our smiling,
our true nature.
Our appointment
with life is in the
present moment.

- THICH NHAT HANH

You may find it easier to practice breathing while lying down. Experiment with resting a book or other light object on your belly, so your arms may rest at your sides.

Renewing your natural breath can take patience. You may find it helpful to write the word *"breathe"* on numerous post-its and place them around your home, car and work place. Strive to pause throughout your day and simply take three deep breaths. Notice how your energy shifts. Feel the difference, before you sit down to eat, prior to preparing food, or with any shift into a new activity.

I encourage you to find the ways that will support you to continually bring your attention to your breath. Breathing habits are not like other exercise habits, which can be practiced in one session at a time. Spending conscious time breathing once a day will not produce the positive result that numerous shorter intervals speckled throughout your day — and a shift in awareness of your breathing all of the time — will.

The more present you are in your breathing, the better. You may wish to repeat the words, *"I am breathing in, I am breathing out."*

It is common for your mind to be somewhere other than on your breathing. We are not accustomed to thinking about our breathing. Be aware that each breath is a gift of life and the more present we are, the more our bodies can receive that gift.

If you enjoy visualizations or affirmations, I encourage you to close your eyes or soften your gaze and bring to mind an image that relaxes you and that can fully occupy your attention while you breathe. Feel the beauty or joy of what you are envisioning. Consider repeating an affirmation aimed to make each breath more potent. *"I release my tension with each exhalation." "I breathe in compassion and understanding." "I am beautiful and youthful."* The possibilities are endless.

There are two breathing exercises with movement that are especially helpful and enjoyable. These can be done once a day or as often as you like.

Heaven & Earth Breath

The Heaven & Earth Breath (*aka Sun Breath*) is deeply balancing and quite wonderful, even more so if you are able to perform it outside.

- Begin by sitting in an upright position. Allow your arms to be loosely by your sides. As you inhale, feel your breath assist you as you "breathe" your arms out to the sides, palms facing down. If possible, continue to bring your arms up overhead until the back of your hands meet. Then rotate your palms to face each other.
- As you exhale, float your arms down with your palms facing upward. The movement of your arms is paced by the length of your breath.
- When you have taken in as much air as you can, your arms should be meeting overhead.
- When you have fully exhaled, your arms will be back by your sides.

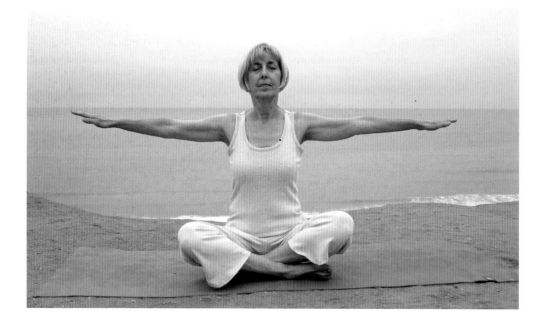

TIP: I find it helpful to close my eyes and imagine the different forces flowing within my body. Try asking yourself: *What would heaven's energy or light look like within your body? How far can you draw this energy or light down into or over your body? How easy is it to draw Earth's energy up into or over your body? What color would each of these energies be? Are you more receptive to one than the other? Can you create a deeper sense of balance within your body?*

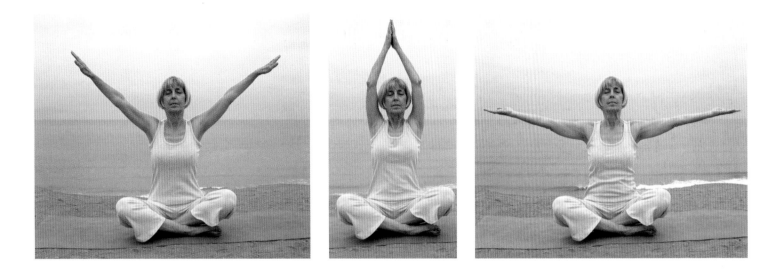

MODIFICATION: Simplify, by bringing your arms to shoulder height. If a physical limitation impedes movement on one side, feel free to use one arm in the exercise, while you visualize the other arm moving. Strive to do what you can, without overdoing. In time, most people can increase their range of motion as they harmonize lifting their arms with their breath. The more we use the power of our breath, the more effortless stretching will be.

As you breathe the arms up, stretch out through every finger, separating them from each other. As you bring your awareness here, know that this awareness helps in extending your stretch. Let your palms be receptive, like sponges. This breath grounds and centers the body and mind.

Imagine, as you are breathing in, that the earth's energy is pushing your arms up. As you exhale, feel heaven's energy shining down, bringing a sense of equilibrium to your whole being. When we harmonize our breathing, our stretching, and our visualizing this way, we can feel an effortless surge of energy. This Heaven & Earth Breath offers us this awareness. It is also used for balancing the masculine and feminine forces within us.

For some people, seeing the breath as a color helps by giving the mind something tangible to focus on. The color can change as the breath moves through or leaves your body. Let your mind help you. Be creative in finding ways to receive the most benefit and energy.

The Heaven & Earth Breath can be repeated seven times, or as often as you like.

Joy of Breath *(aka Breath of Joy and Breath of Life)*

- Begin by sitting or standing in an upright position. You will be taking three full deep inhalations *before* exhaling. The intention is to fill your lungs to capacity with air, and then bend forward to expel the air.
- Inhale and bring your arms out in front of your body.
- Inhale deeply again as you extend your arms to your sides.
- On your third inhalation bring your arms up overhead if possible.
- Then exhale as you fully release forward, bending at your waist.

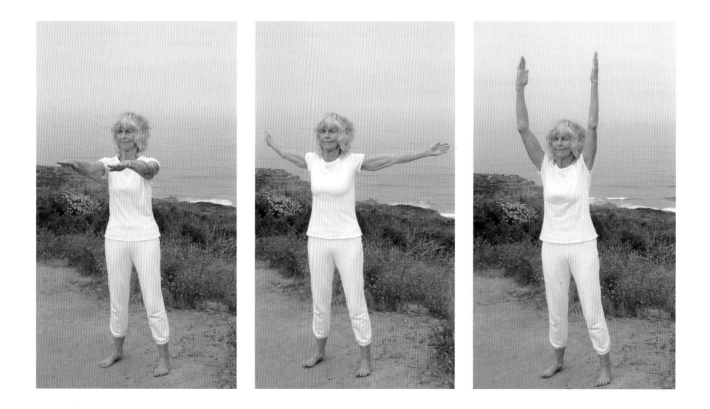

MODIFICATION: If you are standing and wish to protect your lower back, simply bring your hands to your thighs on your exhalation. As you inhale back up, push off of your legs to further support your spine. Work your way up to seven repetitions of this every day if possible. You'll feel warmer and more joyful! This breath helps to expand our lung capacity by releasing stale air.

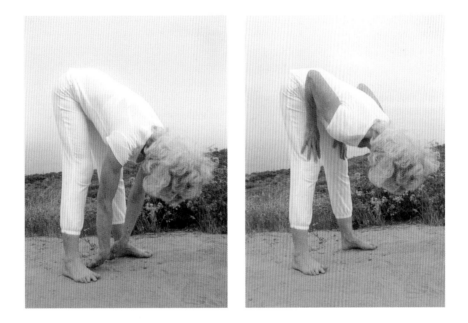

Remind yourself, this moment will not ever happen again.
Drink it in.
Feel the joy of life.
Smile.

Smiling is very important.
If we are not able to smile, then the world will not have peace.
It is with our capacity of smiling, breathing,
and being peace that we can make peace.

~ THICH NHAT HANH

Models: *In order of appearance:*
Donna Jacobsen, 65 youthful years.
Julia Burgess-Perrot, 74 years young.

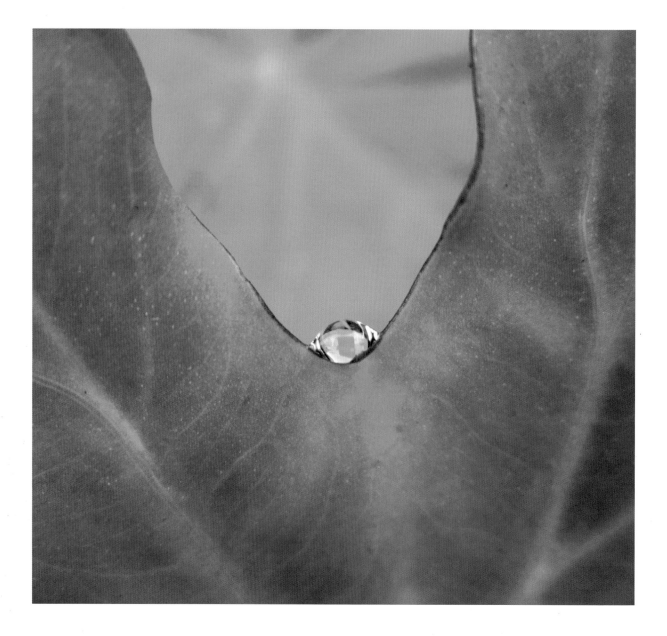

Our bodies communicate to us clearly and specifically,
if we are willing to listen to them.

~ SHAKTI GAWAIN

Do-In:
your medicinal, magical hands

Just What is Do-In?

Do-In (dough-een) is a series of healing, diagnostic and energizing self-massage techniques that originated thousands of years ago in the Far East. This ancient practice is known to increase energy, clarity and well-being in the body, mind and spirit. The discoveries were initially considered to be coveted wisdom and were verbally passed on for generations. By embracing this practice, we take our health and awareness into our own hands.

Do-In exercises are comprised of movements, including tapping, pounding, pinching, pulling and rubbing. They are performed to energize and balance our life force, also known as *chi* or *ki.* Our chi flows through pathways in our body known as meridians. Each meridian relates to an organ or system, and in good health, our chi circulates freely throughout its path. If our chi becomes blocked or stagnated, we may experience sensation, or pain, along the pathway. Blockages can occur for a number of reasons. These common occurrences are the minor aches and pains that we may experience seemingly without explanation.

I discovered Do-In while studying macrobiotic cuisine with its founder, Michio Kushi. One of the life-altering aspects of embracing macrobiotics for me was that we practiced Do-In daily. When I began my studies, I was in my early 20's and the concept of chi was completely foreign to me. However, as I practiced this exercise, with its simple yet powerful techniques, I realized how much lighter and energetic I felt. It was as though a hunger was being deeply satiated in the pre-dawn light at Kushi's macrobiotic summer camps. I didn't understand it then, and some mystery still pervades, though 30 years later, Do-In is part of my daily life.

In short, practicing Do-In helps to regulate and enhance energy flow in the body. The light finger massage techniques can calm excess energy that has become blocked at various points in your body. If there is excess energy at one point, this means there is a shortage somewhere else in your body. As Jacques De Langre, author of *The First Book of Do-In*, published in 1971, explains, "When there is excess energy in a meridian, it is necessary to calm it by dispersing it ... if this is not done, this energy, just like any stagnant water, becomes polluted..."

The exercises can be done by anyone, at any time, and do not require any additional tools or instruments. Reflexology, acupressure, shiatsu and acupuncture all evolved from the ancient practice of Do-In.

The Greater Possibility of Do-In

The original practitioners of Do-In were fueled by a belief that they encompassed more than their individual bodies. They believed that all living things are connected, and that by taking care of themselves they were improving the quality of life everywhere. These creators had a profound understanding and embodiment of energy that we can only vaguely grasp today. Their wellspring of knowledge is a lasting inspiration.

If we too, embrace the belief that the quality of our energy, thoughts and actions influence others, we may be even more inspired to take greater care of ourselves.

Preparing for Your Practice

When you practice Do-In on a daily basis, your body awareness is heightened and you begin to notice subtle changes. In the beginning, you may experience sensation when you press areas, or points, along your body. This light pain will dissipate upon release of the pressure, and over time will usually lessen. When sensation is present in your body it can be an indication of an existing internal condition. It is helpful to experience this sensation, which may indicate a blockage, as an invitation to bring more focused healing touch.

The invitation is about participation, not mere observation. We are not journeying in the universe but with the universe. We are not concerned about living in an evolving world but co-evolving with our world. We are parts of a whole, much greater than the sum of its parts, and yet within each part we are interconnected with the whole.

– DIARMUID O'MURCHU

Similar to yoga, some movements in Do-In replicate animals in their natural habitat. Upon rising, animals innately nourish their bodies through stretching and movement. You may find that you already intuitively do a number of the exercises.

Massage and chi practices are most effective when you invite your intuition to guide your practice. As you deepen your breath and quiet your mind, it will feel as if your body is guiding you. Welcome, with ease and confidence, your natural abilities and divine talents.

This program offers a sampling of the many exercises that are possible. Feel free to create a flow or routine that honors your body and your timeframe. Trust that your body will provide you with feedback about your practice.

All of these exercises can be done from the floor, sitting on a bed, or a chair. What is most important is that you are comfortable, that your posture is upright and your breath is deep.

Use Do-In as an energizing warm-up to any exercise routine. You may feel as though you are warming your body from the inside out! Pause as often as you wish, and delight in the energy you are creating. Enjoy!

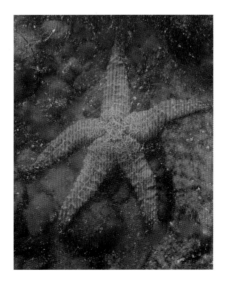

*One can make a day of any size and regulate the rising and
setting of his own sun and the brightness of its shining.*

~ JOHN MUIR

The Practice

WARMING YOUR HANDS

- To begin, take three deep breaths in and out through your nostrils. Rub your hands together vigorously to warm them and strengthen the flow of your energy.

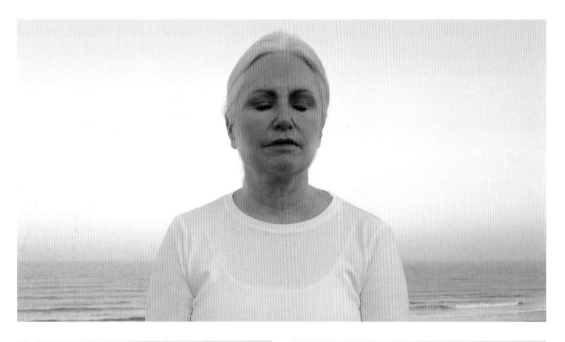

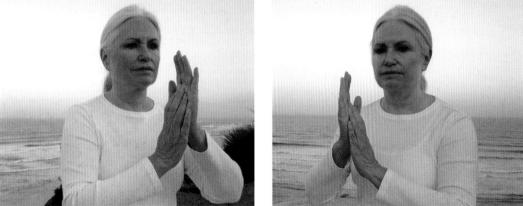

HEAD AND HAIR

These scalp exercises are known to stimulate your brain, affecting both physical and mental activity. They also stimulate your bladder and gall bladder. Often this results in a feeling of being more alert and refreshed. Enjoy these exercises first thing in the morning or any time you feel drowsy.

- Make a fist and pound lightly all over your scalp while keeping your wrist loose.
- With your fingertips, rub your scalp vigorously.
- Gather fistfuls of hair and pull on them gently. For those with very short hair, grasp even a few hairs, and pull gently with intention.

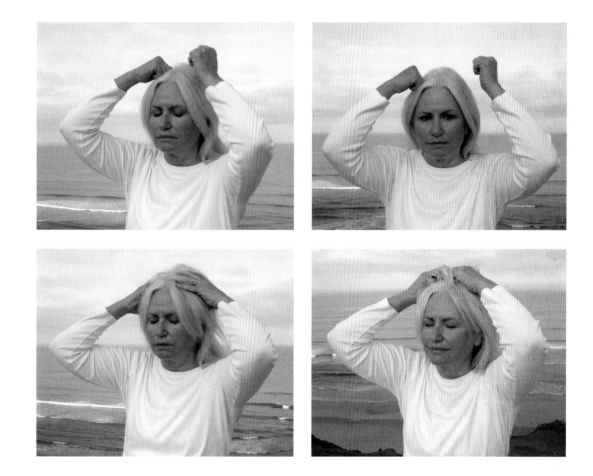

FACE

These facial exercises are effective for releasing tension. You may instinctively do some of these exercises when you have a headache; doing them regularly and proactively can help prevent headaches and keep you relaxed.

- With your fingertips tap gently all over your forehead. Close your eyes and take your time, moving gradually, as you feel the tension releasing. Let your body guide you.
- Tap your temples.
- Gently rub your temples in a circular motion using the tips of your fingers.
- Gently pinch your eyebrows, lightly pull forward and then release. Begin at the bridge of your nose and work out toward your temples.

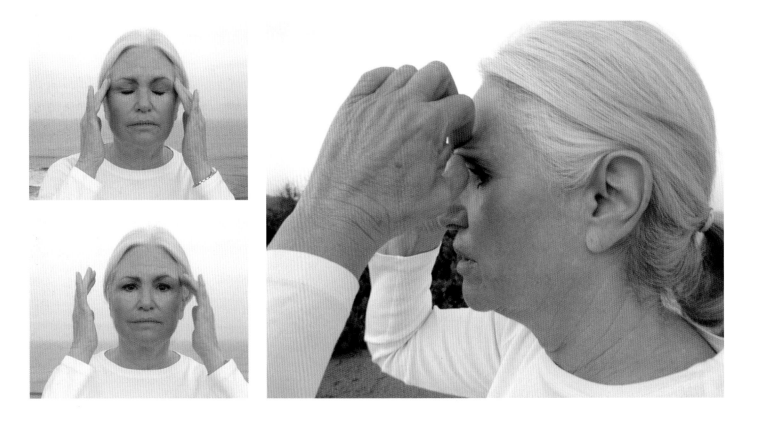

NOSE

The nose is the gateway to the lungs. Do-In exercises for the nose can help maintain clear sinus passageways and lessen symptoms of colds and flus.

- With your thumb and forefinger, firmly pinch and release the tip of your nose three times.
- Pinch midway up your nose three times and release.
- Pinch the bridge of your nose, holding for about 10 seconds. Then release and repeat three times. This point is called "Clear Brightness." It is believed that this exercise promotes clear vision.
- With your index fingers, rub the sides of your nose until you feel warmth. Begin at the base and rub upward. This is especially helpful if you have been in heavy pollution and wish to clear your sinus pathways. This exercise also energizes the stomach and pancreas.

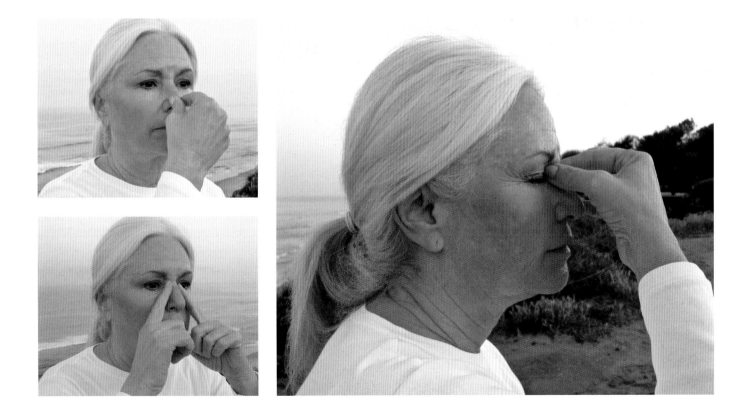

EYES

There are many eye exercises to strengthen your eyes, improve your vision and help to correct or eliminate concerns with the eyes. It is believed that the eyes and liver meridian are connected. As we strengthen the liver, our eyesight will be strengthened. Conversely, if concerns arise with the eyes it can be an indication of a need to strengthen the liver.

- Begin by rubbing your palms together to re-warm them. Feel free to warm them throughout this exercise.
- Rest your fingers over your closed eyelids for as long as it is comfortable. With your eyes still closed, look up as far you can, and then down as far as you can.
- Continue, looking as far left and as far right as you can. Diagonally, look to your upper right and then to your lower left. Move on to making circles clockwise and then afterward, counterclockwise.
- Remember to breathe deeply. Gradually build up to ten repetitions of these eye stretches.

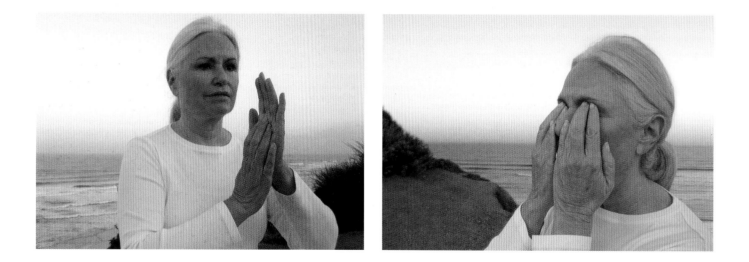

- With your fingertips, apply a firm and focused pressure near the bridge of your nose and upper corner of the eye socket. Hold for several seconds. Next, apply pressure on the base of the eye socket toward the inside. Then repeat the pressure closer to the temple.

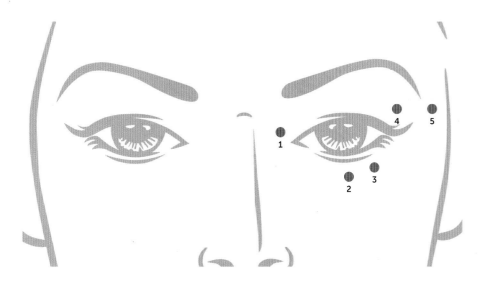

- Now press on the outer upper eye socket.
- Finally, press near the temple and outside edge of the socket.
- Repeat these movements three times in the direction described. (Reversing the direction can produce a tiring effect.)
- With your fingertips, trace lightly along the bones of your eye sockets. Begin at the bridge, on the inside and simultaneously press your finger up toward your eyebrow, then out toward your temples, down, and back in toward your nose. Move your fingers in a clockwise direction around your right eye and counter-clockwise around your left eye. Do not reverse.

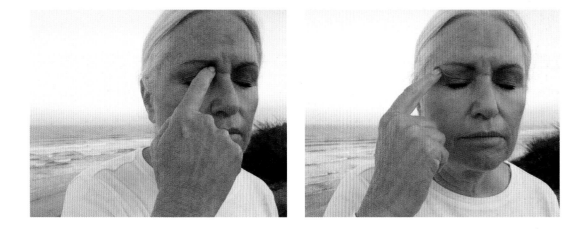

CHEEKS

Many people find great release from these two simple cheek exercises.

- Tap all over your cheeks with your fingertips. This can help energize your breathing, clear your sinuses and release tension.
- Apply deep pressure up under the cheekbone. Repeat three times to stimulate your stomach meridian.

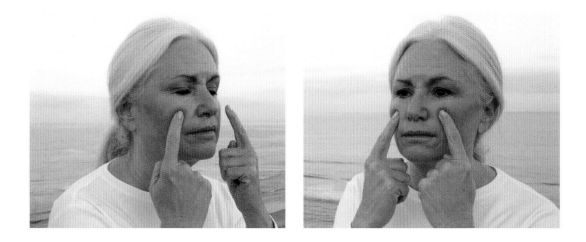

JAW & MOUTH

The jaw and the mouth are important areas to focus on. The jaw holds more tension than most people realize.

- With your fingertips, gently rub in a circular motion where the upper and lower jaw meet in front of the ear.
- Continue circular rubbing along your top gum line toward the center, and then back to your jaw. Repeat for your bottom gums.

Rubbing your gums nourishes vitality of the gums and of the meridians that connect with every tooth. You may wish to incorporate this practice into your daily dental hygiene. Every one of your teeth is connected to an organ.

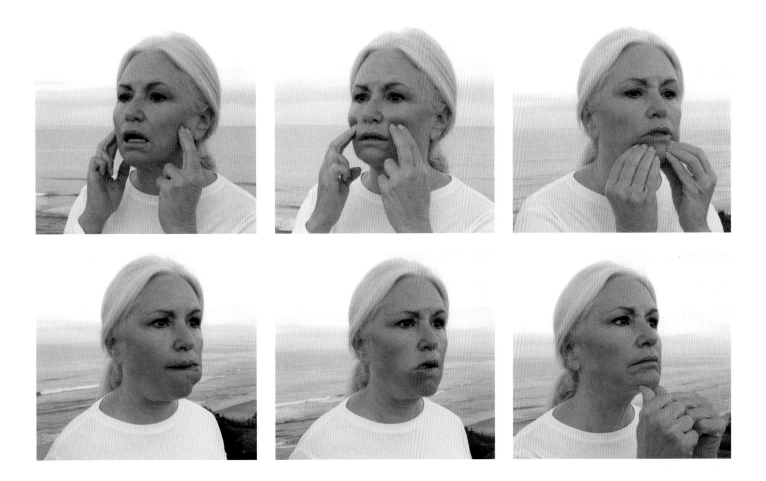

Just as the eyes can be an indication of an underlying concern with the liver, the teeth are a roadmap to your body. Whole body dental charts are available online and from biological dentists. I encourage you to learn more about the important connection of your teeth to your overall health. See *naomicall.com* for more information

- Roll your tongue over your teeth and gums. This action produces saliva and stimulates the heart muscles. The tongue is considered to be the opening to the heart. The Chinese refer to saliva as "heavenly water." Saliva helps to eliminate germs and aids digestion.
- Massage the thumbs underneath the chin to help prevent a sagging double chin.

EARS

The ears are believed to be the gateway to the kidneys. Do-In ear exercises also stimulate the pineal gland, which is connected to, and in line with the ears. The pineal gland is referred to as the center of spiritual awareness.

- Pull and stretch the ears in all directions.

Pulling down on the lobes is said to create "happiness and serenity." Many people discover that they enjoy massaging their ears and having them massaged more than they would have imagined. They also report feeling more centered and tranquil afterward.

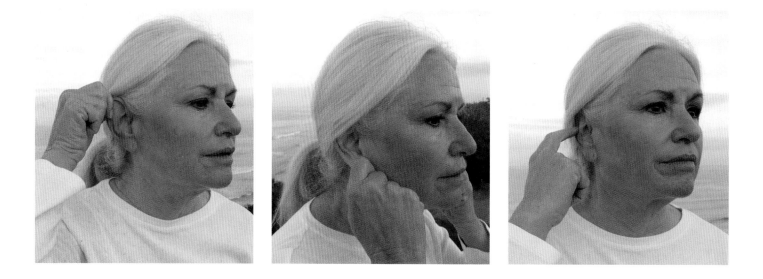

- With your index finger, gently trace from the center of your ear, following the curve if the outer ear. Repeat three times.
- Fold your outer ear over, closing off your ear and then release. Repeat three times. Lightly tap on your ears with your opposite hand while your ear is folded over. This is called "Beating the Heavenly Drum."

The ear is often overlooked. There are over one hundred acupuncture points in the ears that are easily energized with light touch.

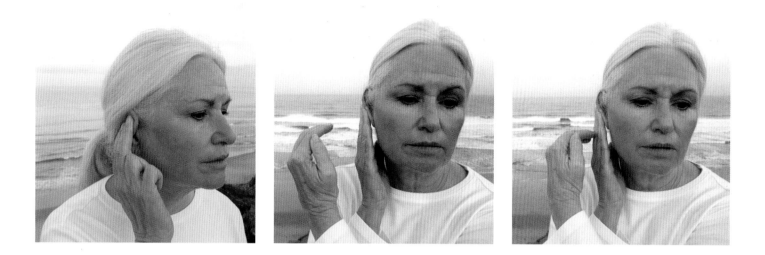

ARMS AND HANDS

• With a loose wrist, pound your fist along the ridge of your shoulders and lower neck.

Many people hold tension here. Take your time, and extra deep breaths. The large intestine and triple heater meridians are located on the shoulder ridge. The triple heater governs circulation and sexual energy.

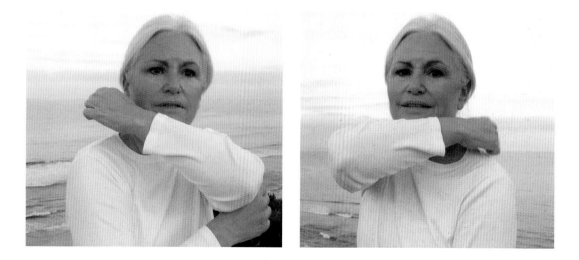

- Press your fingers deeply into your shoulder ridge. Then grip and rotate your shoulder joint.
- Gently pound down your arms from your shoulder to your wrists. Keep your wrists loose. Then, squeeze and release your arms, beginning at the shoulder, and working your way down to the wrist. This exercise circulates energy to the heart, small and large intestines, triple heater and heart governor meridians.

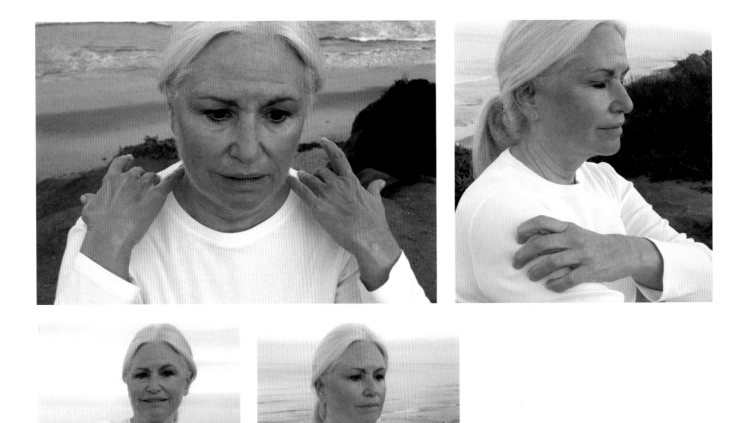

- Shake your wrists, first with your palms facing up, and then, with your palms down. Now flick your wrists from side to side.

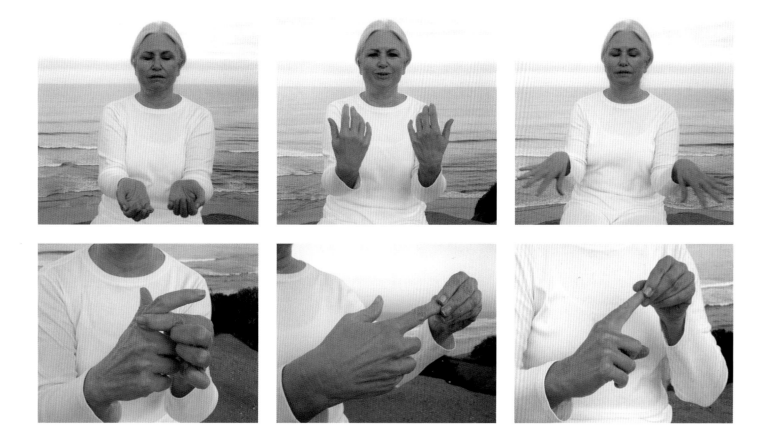

The most important acupressure points are located around the wrist. Maintain a flexible wrist throughout your practice. This will energize and tone your lungs, intestines, circulation and sexual energy.

- Begin at the base of each finger working your way to the tip. Massage the sides of each finger with your opposite index finger and thumb. Then pull the tip and release it quickly. Take each finger and rotate it. Meridians run along the *sides* of your fingers.

- Notice the union of the index and thumb. Press your opposite thumb up and under the point where these two supporting bones join. Rub in a deep, circular motion. This point is often sensitive. Deeply massage 3 - 5 seconds throughout your day for improved colon function and overall health. Many acupuncturists consider this a key point for longevity. If pregnant, please avoid massaging here.
- With your fingertips, massage around the inside base of the thumb to nourish your lung and large intestine.
- Gently press each finger as far back as possible. Take your time stretching each finger in both directions. Experiment with using your opposite fingers or palm to see what works best for you.

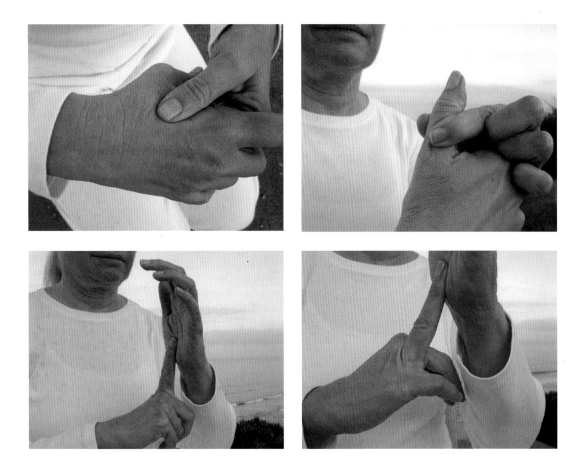

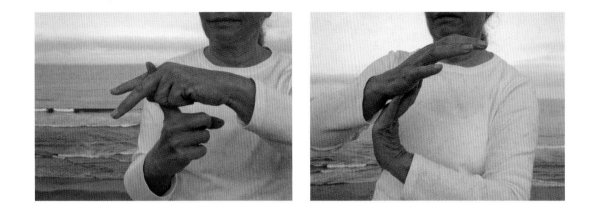

When you release each finger, an extra boost of energy moves through your meridian.

- Next, bend all of the fingers back at one time and release. Bend the thumbs back and release.

A sign of good health is demonstrated by achieving a 90-degree angle as you press your fingers backward. Be patient.

- With your thumb and index finger, pinch and quickly release both sides of the tip of your opposite baby finger. Repeat 3 - 5 times. Stimulating this point is known for diminishing heart attacks.
- Another point for heart health is located on the palm below the baby finger. Gently rub with all fingers in a circular motion for 3 - 5 seconds.

TIP: A student shared that her physician told her that if she thought she was having a heart attack to bite down on both of her baby fingers!

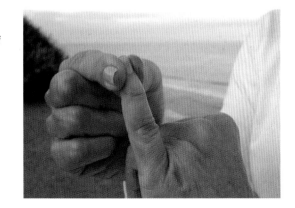

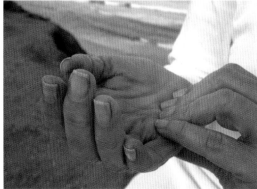

- Flex and rotate your wrists.
- Then, stretch your thumb across your palm to the *base, not the tip,* of your baby finger. Follow by stretching every other finger across to the *base* of the thumb.
- It is naturally difficult to isolate the baby finger in a stretch; your other fingers will want to follow!
- Repeat the exercise with the other hand. Pause and feel the warmth in your hands.

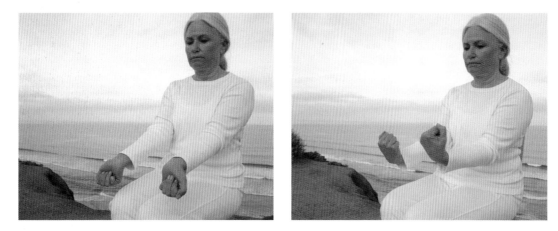

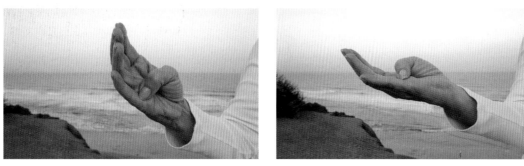

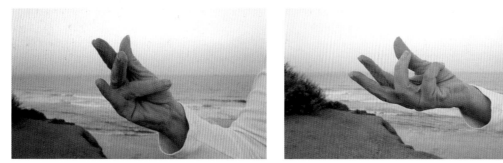

- Clasp your fingers and wiggle them around. Then, gradually pull your hands apart while continuing to wiggle your fingers. Repeat the exercise with the opposite thumb and fingers on top.
- Circle your thumbs three times in one direction, then repeat in the opposite direction.

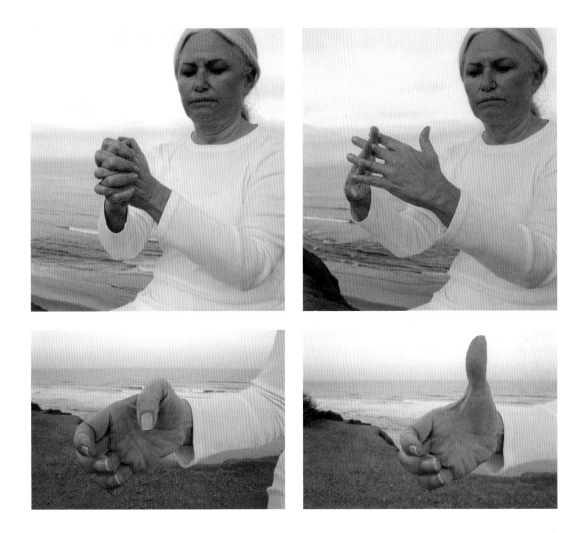

Most people experience greater circulation in their fingers after practicing these exercises. Dexterity can be enhanced when these are done with regularity.

CHEST AND UPPER TORSO

Do-In chest exercises help to release stagnation in the lymphatic system, strengthen the respiratory function and accelerate blood flow. A sense of warmth and itchiness is a sign that you have activated chi flow.

- With your fingertips, tap all around your chest, especially the sternum. Tapping on your sternum is often helpful for awakening and centering yourself.
- Lightly pound and rub with your fingertips all over the chest. Rub lightly in between the ribs, this may be a little sensitive.

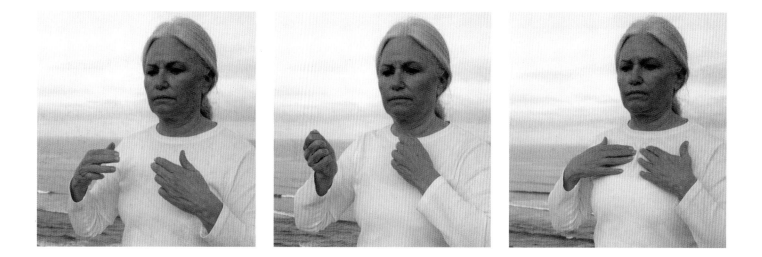

Especially for women who do *not* have breast cancer, taking a few moments to massage your breasts can help facilitate the release of tenderness due to accumulated energy. These regularly occurring blockages of energy are usually related to diet, lifestyle or emotions. Massaging the breasts is an easy preventative breast health measure. This will often result in a feeling of being lighter and clearer. For women who have had, or currently have breast cancer, massage is usually not recommended. (See Sex and Longevity chapter for more breast health tips.)

- Vigorously rub the sides of your rib cage. This action stimulates the liver and spleen meridians. Press your fingers up under your right rib cage, massaging and nourishing the liver. Then do the same on the left side, where the spleen is located.

TIP: Hot water bottles are soothing to the belly, and can strengthen digestive forces. You may wish to cover your bottle with a flannel pillowcase and enjoy the comforting effects while reading or watching television.

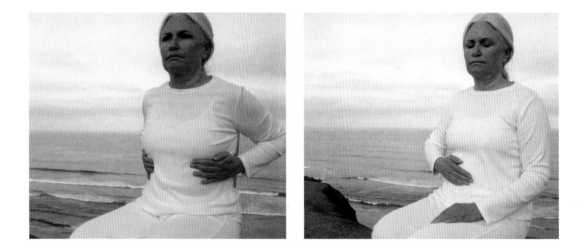

- Massage the abdominal area in a clockwise motion with one or both hands. This exercise soothes and calms while also aiding in digestion.

BACK & BUTTOCKS

- Place your hands on the lower back area, over the kidneys and adrenals. Lift up and stretch back slowly as you take in a deep breath. Hold for two more breaths. Option: Release and soften forward with your exhalation. Repeat as desired.

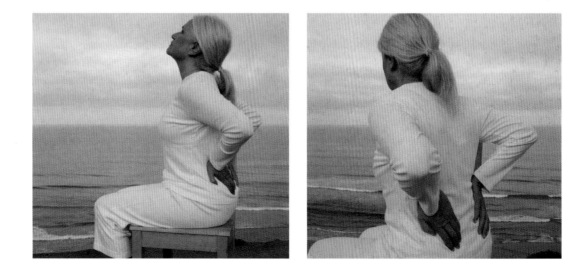

- With a fist, pound gently on your back, as far up and down as you can comfortably reach. This exercise generates energy flow through the kidney, spleen, liver, gall bladder and bladder meridians. It is important to go gently over the kidney area. You can also vigorously rub instead.
- From standing, or a gentle squat, pound all over the buttocks. This tends to be a stagnant area on most people! Feel free to pound more aggressively here.

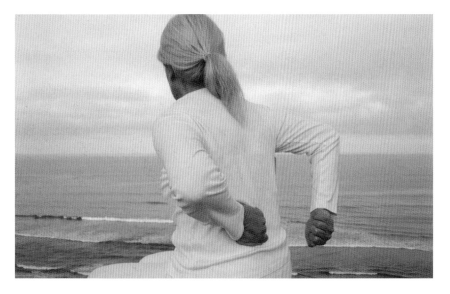

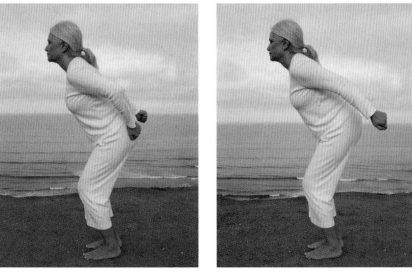

LEGS AND FEET

Meridians do not flow in a straight line, though they do have definite paths. The stomach meridian flows down the front of the leg from the knee to the top of the foot, toward your second and third toe. The spleen meridian flows along the inside of the leg from the knee to the top of the foot. The liver meridian also flows on the inside of the leg and then toward the big toe. The bladder meridian flows along the back of the leg ending at the baby toe. The gall bladder meridian flows down the front of the thigh toward the outside of the leg and ends at the fourth toe.

- Massage, or gently pound down the outside of your legs.

The meridians for the gall bladder, bladder and stomach are all located toward the outside of your legs. This exercise can help to alleviate conditions such as high blood pressure, obesity, and water retention.

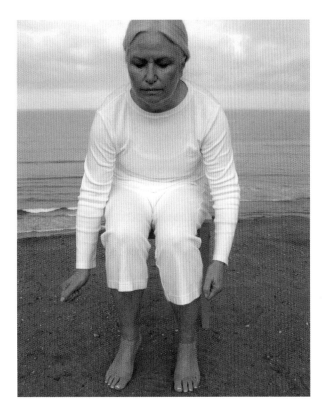

- Massage, or gently rub upward, the inside of your legs.

The meridians that regulate the kidneys, the liver and the pancreas are located on the inside of your legs. This exercise helps to stimulate circulation throughout the lower body. Increased blood flow can help to reduce or eliminate varicose veins and leg cramps. Repeat the leg exercises three times. If you currently have varicose veins, start gently and increase pressure slowly over time as your condition improves.

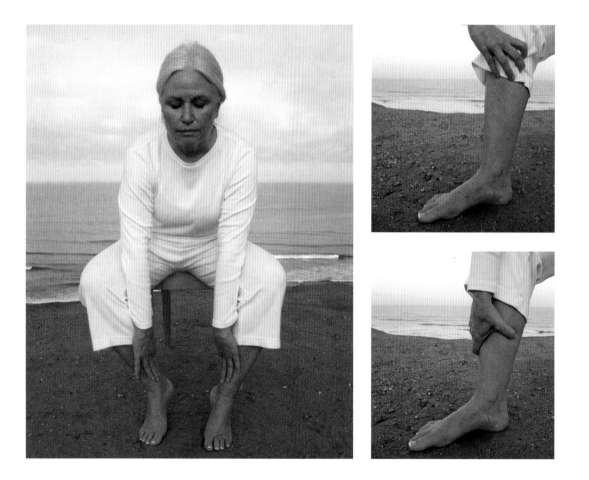

REMINDER: Follow your intuition. If you are drawn to squeeze or more deeply massage your calves, take time to follow your body's lead. If there is tenderness, take an extra deep breath. The next time you do these exercises, pay attention to changes in how you feel.

- Squeeze and massage the knee-cap to loosen tension and increase energy flow throughout your leg.
- Shake a Leg! Pick up your leg and give it a shake.

Usually, your mind will want to move your foot. In this exercise, let your foot be completely relaxed, then vigorously shake your leg! It's eye-opening to see how we often hold tension in parts of our body without realizing it. This exercise can stimulate circulation throughout your body.

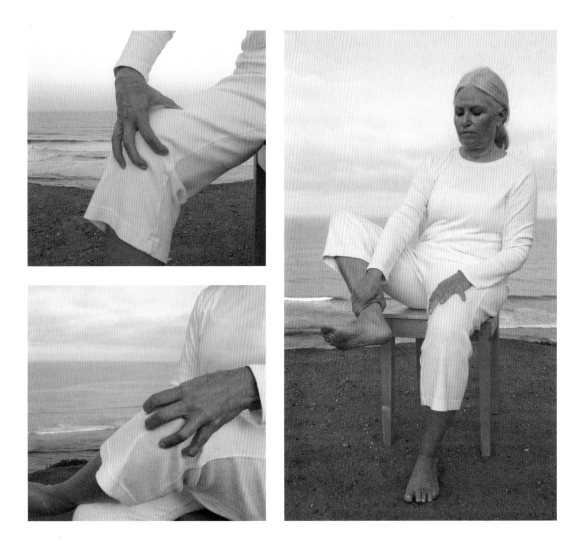

- If possible, rest your foot on your thigh, or modify by bending over to reach your feet. With a loose wrist, pound your fist all over your foot. Or, you might prefer to slap or tap with the fingers.

Stimulating your feet offers a feeling of overall rejuvenation. There are numerous points on our feet that connect to every part of our body. Our feet support us all day and deserve to luxuriate in being touched!

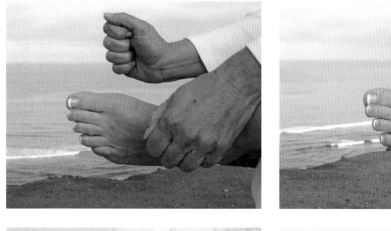

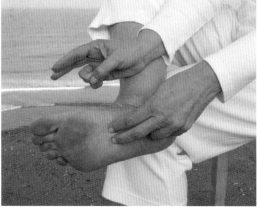

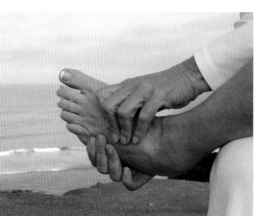

TIP: One student who cannot reach her feet with her hands uses one foot to pound, rub and warm the other foot while she is lying in bed. The activity and stretch also benefit the foot that is delivering the massage.

- Massage the sole of your foot, as deeply as possible, with your knuckles or fingers. Pay extra attention to the arch of your foot.
- Massage your knuckles behind your toes while your cradle your toes with the opposite hand.

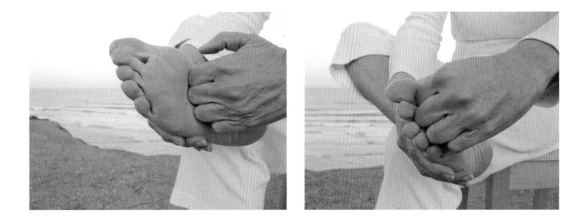

- Massage each toe along its sides, starting at the base. Then pull and release the tip of each toe.

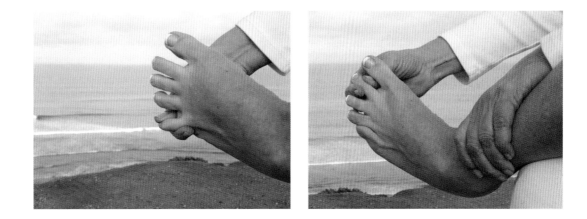

- Wedge all of your fingers in between your toes at the same time. This is often a lively stretch, with a lot of "sensation" being activated. If you are able to wedge your fingers in between, wiggle them around.
  Experiment with working your fingers in from the top of your foot and from the sole to see which is easier. Take a deep breath, then enjoy how good it feels when you pull your fingers out. This is one of my favorites!
- Take a moment to notice how energized your toes feel now!

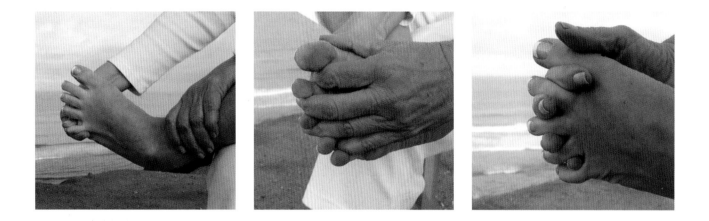

- Press each toe forward and backward. Or stretch them all at once.
- Place your thumb on top of your foot, between the big toe and the second toe. Massage in a circular motion for 5 seconds. Then squeeze the sides of the big toe.
- These exercises stimulate the liver and the spleen.

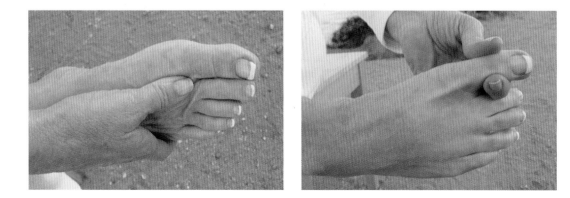

- Massage and pinch down the Achilles tendon. This will stimulate the kidney and the bladder meridians, as well as the testes or ovaries. Then take hold of the heel and work your fingers deeply in to the sole around the heel to further activate your sex glands. This exercise is also known to help ease backaches.

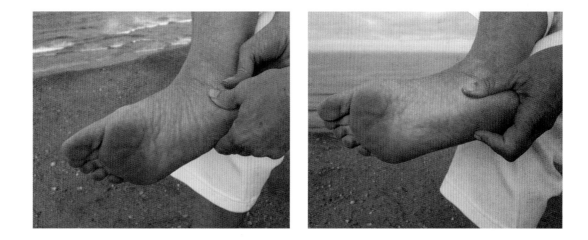

- In a sitting position, lean back and lightly pound your heels on the floor or on your bed. This exercise is known for stimulating bone cell regeneration.

TIP: It is a healthful and precious gift to massage someone else's feet. I encourage you to enliven time with your family and friends by massaging their feet. Even a few minutes while relaxing and watching television can be a delight and leave everyone happier.

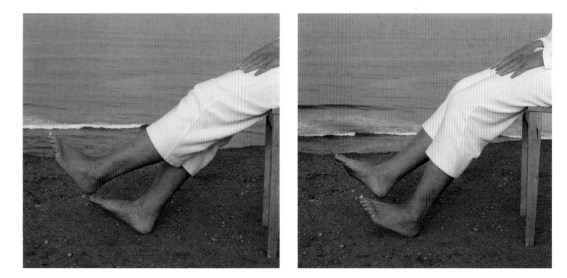

After you have exercised one foot, compare how it feels with your other foot. Notice also how it looks. Pause, and absorb the difference that you have made in a few short moments. Repeat on the other foot.

After you have exercised both feet, pause again, and feel the difference in your whole body. Close your eyes and take in three deep breaths.

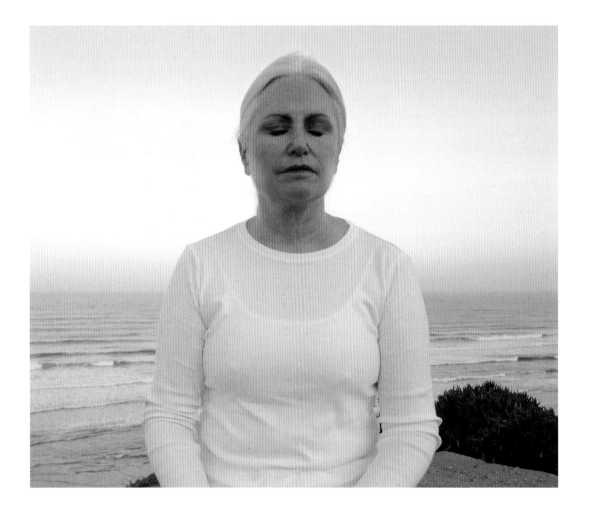

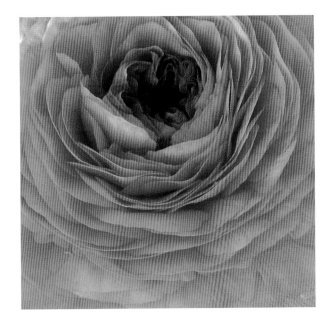

Know thyself.

~ INSCRIBED IN GOLD ON
APOLLO'S TEMPLE
AT DELPHI

Model: *Patty Arambarri,*
Do-In student and model
is 65 years young.

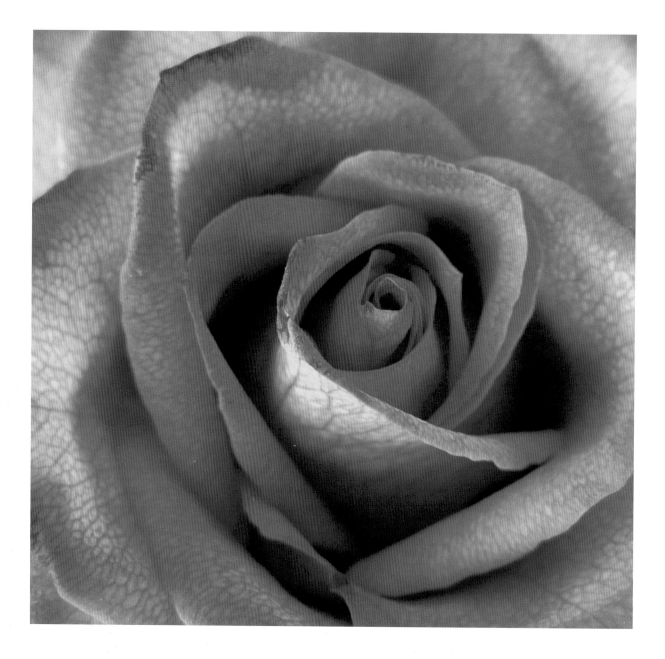

What we think, we become.

— *BUDDHA*

The Five Rites:
"the ancient secret to
the fountain of youth"

The Five Rites were first introduced to Western culture by Peter Kelder in his book, *The Eye of the Revelation*. Published originally in 1939, the book was revised nearly fifty years later, and re-titled *The Ancient Secret of the Fountain of Youth*.

I became intrigued by the idea of these "fountain of youth exercises" over twenty years ago when my mother began practicing them. The continued widespread interest in the Rites can be attributed to the power of the mind, our human fascination with the concept of agelessness, and the Rites' accessibility. These exercises can tone, energize and strengthen all the major muscle groups, organs, chakras and systems in the body.

How the Rites Came To Be

In his book, Mr. Kelder shares the story of his good fortune in learning of these exercises. His discovery began one day while sitting in the park, where he met a man he calls Colonel Bradford. A retired British Army officer, Bradford was in his sixties and had traveled throughout the world, gaining access to very remote areas. The two men shared a lively conversation each time they met. After many meetings, the Colonel revealed that among the people he had heard about in his travels were a group of Lamas in India who were revered for having the "secret to the fountain of youth." He had decided he would return to India to try and find their isolated monastery.

Four years later, Bradford returned to visit Mr. Kelder, and he looked unrecognizably youthful. As he explained to Kelder, persistence and arduous travel resulted in the Colonel finding the Himalayan monastery that was cut off from the outside world. He took up residence there, and now, upon his return, was brimming with stories about his experiences.

Life at the monastery was one of pristine beauty and healthful daily living. The monks walked up steep mountainsides, grew their own food and lived with joy and balance in the fullness of their daily life. The air and the earth that surrounded them was some of the purest on the Earth. These monks, similar to the creators of Do-In, also believed that their efforts of self -improvement were energetically felt and realized far beyond the monastery. They, too, believed that all of life is connected. Even from their remote location, they knew that they were making a widespread difference in the quality of all life on Earth.

Chakras

The first thing the Colonel said that he learned from the monks was that there are seven energy centers, also known as *chakras*, in our body. These centers are linked to our endocrine system and were believed to be a foundation to longevity.

A chakra is a vortex of spinning energy that influences the muscles, organs and systems within its energy field. This concept is relatively new to the West, even though many cultures in the East, especially mystics, have held this belief as a reality for thousands of years. In a healthy body, the energy spins fast; in a body that is weaker, the energy slows down. The belief is that if one of the energy centers in the body slows down, it affects the overall flow of our life force, also known as *prana*. This slowing-down can result in illness and premature aging. Many people believe that one of the fastest ways to youthfulness and vitality is to maintain the normal speed of your chakras spinning. This is due in part to the belief that chakras also influence our endocrine system.

Beliefs about the exact location of the chakras have varied slightly. Generally, the first chakra is located near the perineum or coccyx, the second near the ovaries or prostate, the third near the navel or solar plexus, the fourth near the heart and thymus, the fifth near the thyroid gland, the sixth near the pineal gland or third eye and the seventh near the top of the head. Some people believe there can be as many as ten chakras in the body.

Bradford described to Mr. Kelder how he learned from the monks a series of daily exercises, The Five Rites, which work to keep one's chrakas moving and strong. Even if you find it difficult to embrace the idea of an invisible life force, or prana, in your body, I encourage you to be open-minded and embrace these exercises knowing that rebalancing and strengthening the chakras is only one of the many benefits attributed to the Rites. We will most likely never know for certain if the Colonel's story is entirely true. What we do know is that thousands of people have been performing these exercises and recognizing an improvement in their health and vitality, thanks to Mr. Kelder's initiative.

Preparing for the Exercises

Four of the Rites were originally created for people who are able to get down on the ground. I have developed modifications so that they may be performed using a combination of: the top of your bed, a chair and standing. I work with a wide variety of people, from chronic pain patients to elderly students who use these modifications with ease. I encourage you to be creative in finding the perfect approach for you. As always, only perform what feels right in your body. Yoga and exercise should not hurt.

With every exercise, and every day, conscious breath awareness enriches your outcome. It is best to initially find a quiet spot where you can easily focus on harmonizing your breath. Wear comfortable, loose-fitting clothing. If you are going to be down on the ground, you will need a mat or non-slip padding. Ideally, these exercises are performed in bare feet.

The monks approached exercising by gently building their practice. They slowly added repetitions of an exercise week by week. The Colonel recommended that each Rite be performed three times a day in the first week and increase the repetitions by two each week. At this rate, a person could work up to 21 repetitions in 10 weeks. I find that many people can begin the first week with a goal of working up to 7 repetitions. Then, increase to 14 repetitions the second week. Possibly, by the third week, 21 repetitions are performed. You'll be modifying this to fit your body. Some of the Rites may be more challenging than others.

Often, when I first share the number 21 with people, they react with self-doubt in their ability to accomplish that many. Maintain an open mind, you may find that these exercises flow more quickly and with less effort than anticipated. An energizing routine can easily be performed within fifteen minutes.

Following the original routine as published by Mr. Kelder, I have also provided a modified order for greater ease if you are using your bed or a chair to perform the routine. You may wish to begin with the simplified routine and work your way into the original Rites.

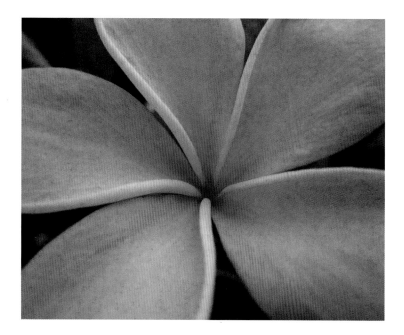

The Rites in Practice

THE FIRST RITE

The act of simply spinning one's physical body is something that most children have done playfully for as long as we can remember. Many forms of dance from Whirling Dervishes to contemporary steps are accentuated and enhanced with spinning one's body.

The first Rite is Spinning, and this is done to re-align, energize and speed up the spinning of the chakras in the body. If you have not spun since you were a young child, I encourage you to *begin very slowly*. Perform only one revolution, stop and make certain that you are not dizzy.

Spinning is always done clockwise. In other words, you will be spinning to your right. Dancers, or people who are familiar with having an eye-level focal point will want to use this technique. Otherwise, some people experiment with raising their right index finger and using their finger as a focal point.

- Stand up straight, have a sense of lifting your spine up out of your waist. Center your weight on the soles of your feet, bring a gentle bend to your knees and slightly tuck your tailbone under. Bring your awareness to your breath.
- Pause, taking three deep breaths to center yourself, and bring your full attention to this moment. Inhale, as you lift your arms out to your sides at shoulder height.
- Begin to slowly rotate clockwise, in other words, to your right. Modify by fixing your gaze onto the tip of your right index finger if this helps you to focus.

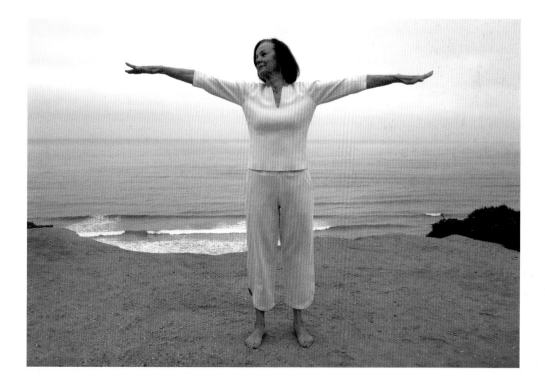

If you are dizzy or light-headed, pause, and resume at another time. If you feel nauseous, even though it feels unpleasant, it is actually helpful to vomit. It is believed that spinning can gather toxicity from the body and it is natural for the body to seek a way to expel it. If you simply go slow, this usually does not happen. If it does, sitting still will also help the feeling to dissipate.

- After you have completed your revolutions, pause, and again take three deep breaths. This enables your body to fully receive the benefit of your movement.

THE SECOND RITE

The second Rite is performed lying on your back on the ground or on your bed.
A number of modifications are offered to honor and protect your spine.

- Begin with deepening your breath. Inhale as you lengthen your arms to your sides with your palms facing down.
- With your next inhalation, lift your head off of the mat or bed as you slowly raise your legs as straight as possible.
- As you exhale, gently release your head and legs down. Pause, and take three deep breaths. Allow the muscles to relax.
- Build your repetitions, as you are able.

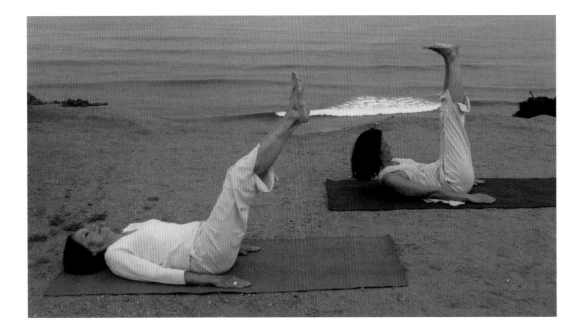

Some people find this to be a challenging Rite; it takes core strength and a strong spine. I encourage you to be patient and take your time strengthening your core. Week by week, add as many repetitions as you are comfortable with. You may find that your abdomen is toned in a short period of time! As we strengthen our core abdominal area and trim extra pounds, we are also greatly supporting the spine.

There are a number of beneficial modifications you can explore while building your core strength.

MODIFICATION ONE: If you have past or present neck injuries, simply lift and lower your legs, keeping your head down. Soften your knees, bending as needed.

MODIFICATION TWO: Simplify by lifting one of your legs until you can lift both legs at once.

MODIFICATION THREE: If it is uncomfortable to lay flat with your legs straight, experiment with adding a cushion under your knee to support your spine.

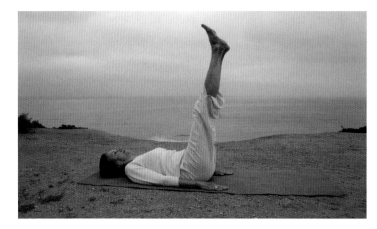
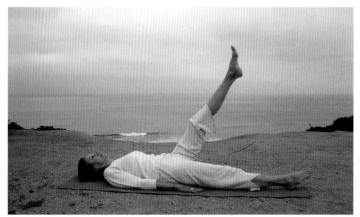

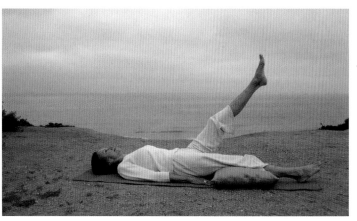

CORE STRENGTHENING REPLACEMENT EXERCISE:

If you have neck concerns, or find it too difficult to raise your legs, you may find this to be a good replacement for the second Rite. In yoga, this would be likened to a modified boat pose.

- Rest on your tailbone, with your knees bent. Lengthen your arms along the sides of your body, parallel with the earth.
- As you inhale, lengthen your legs out as far as you can comfortably, while softening your spine toward the ground or your bed.
- Exhale, and draw your body back up and into your starting position.

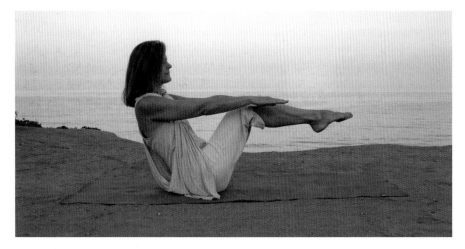

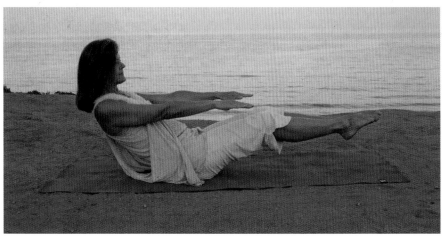

THE THIRD RITE

This Rite can be done on the ground, on a padded chair or on your bed.

- Begin by taking deep breathes. Bring your body into an upright position on your knees with your toes curled under. If you are on the ground, place the palms of your hands on the back of your thighs.
- Exhale, as you tuck your chin to your chest and round your spine. Inhale, as you lift up and stretch your spine back, drawing your shoulder blades together. Strive to develop an awareness of an invisible thread that runs from your tailbone to the top of your head. Imagine that someone is lifting you up with that thread.
- Press your hands into your thighs or buttocks, whichever one is more supportive.
- Take three deep breaths upon completion. Repeat as desired.

MODIFICATION: If performing this Rite on your bed, a headboard can be very helpful to hold onto, instead of your thighs. You can also use the back of a chair in the same way.

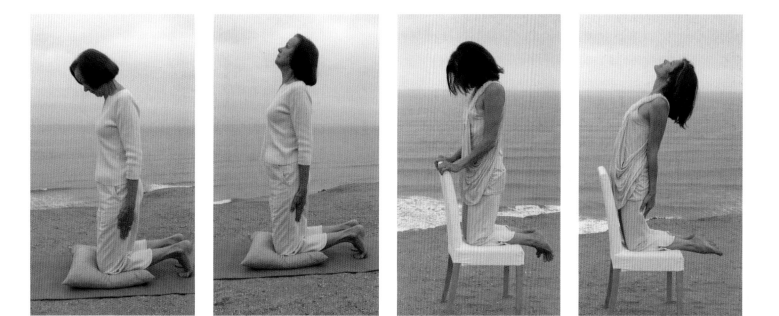

THE FOURTH RITE

This Rite can be done on the ground or on your bed.

* Begin by sitting with your spine lifted. Lengthen your legs as straight as possible in front of you, with your feet about 12 inches apart. Place your palms beside your buttocks with your fingertips pointing toward your feet.
* As you inhale, draw the crown of your head back as you raise your belly toward the ceiling or sky.
* As you exhale, draw your lower torso down. Ideally, your hips and tailbone will glide between your hands and your heels will not move. Keep your feet planted in the same place.

The goal is to bring your back and body, parallel to the floor or your bed. Similar to a porch glider, your body flows up, and then glides back through. This may take time and patience. This exercise utilizes our upper-body strength.

* Repeat as desired. Pause for three deep breaths.

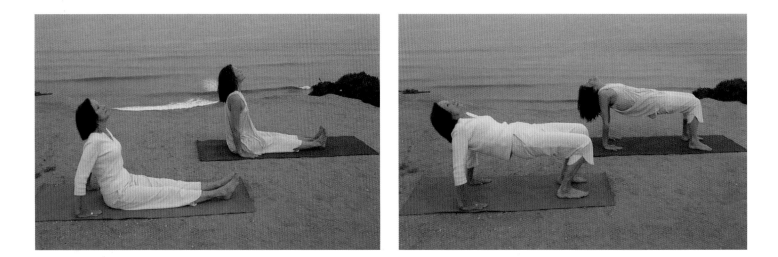

MODIFICATIONS: You may wish to experiment with your fingertips pointing away from your body. Go gently. In the beginning, you might only lift your body an inch or two off of the ground. Visualize your body being all the way up!

THE FIFTH RITE

This Rite is performed on the ground, either with or without a chair. It can be simply modified to be one of the easier Rites to perform. Take a deep breath before you begin.

IF ON A MAT.
- Begin on your belly. As you inhale, lift your body up off of the mat with your toes curled under. Keep a gentle bend in your elbows, and your shoulders soft as you press the crown of your head toward the sky, and then back.

IF USING A CHAIR.
- Create space between you and your chair. As you inhale, lift your heart to the heavens as you press your hips toward the chair. Squeeze your shoulder blades back and together. You may wish to stretch your toes up off of the ground.

In yoga, this position is known as the upward dog.

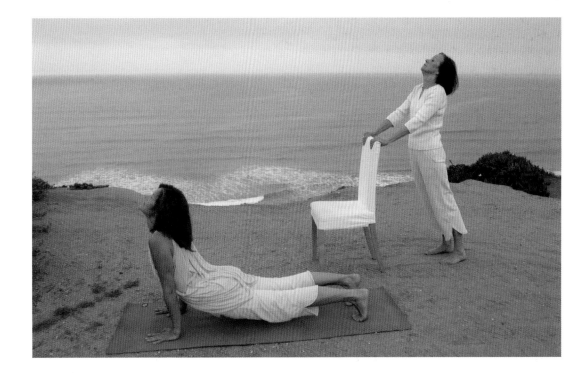

IF ON A MAT.

- As you exhale, press your hips toward the sky as you tuck your chin. Press your tail-bone back to increase a stretch in the hamstrings. Ease your heels toward the mat, or visualize them touching.

IF USING A CHAIR.

- As you exhale, press your tailbone back toward the wall or space behind you. Keep your knees gently soft as you fold forward. Let your head drop between your arms.

This position is known as the downward dog. Repeat as desired. Take three deep breaths.

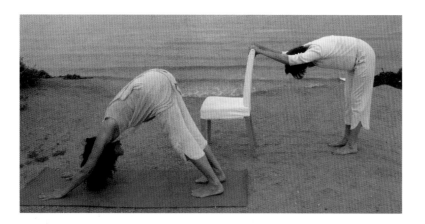

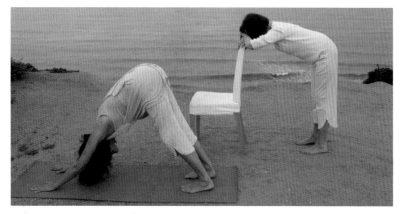

MODIFICATION: Experiment with adjusting the distance of your body to your chair. Consider resting your forearms on the back of your chair, instead of extending your arms. Then, you can rest your forehead on your forearms.

Simplifying the Routine

You may wish to explore performing the Rites in a modified order for ease of movements. This order works well for many people:

- Begin standing with Rite 1.
- Next, lay down on your back for Rite 2. Then roll onto your side and come into a sitting position.
- Now, onto Rite 4. When complete roll onto your belly or come into a standing position.
- Follow with Rite 5.
- Finish on your knees with Rite 3.

Feel free to modify the order to honor and create a flow that is right for your body. It is preferable to do even a few of each one. Remember to pause and breathe.

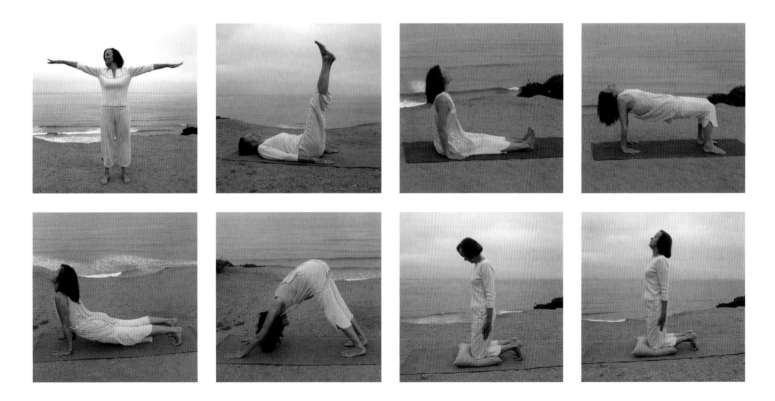

OPTION: There is also a variation of the Rites that advocates a complete pause in between each Rite, by moving into a pose known as the Child. Simply taking in three deep breaths in between each Rite is sufficient for your body to receive the benefit of your efforts and enables you to stay in a more fluid flow.

Pictured below is the yoga pose known as the Child, if you wish to explore this addition to your practice. There are a number of variations to this pose, which is also described in the Yoga chapter.

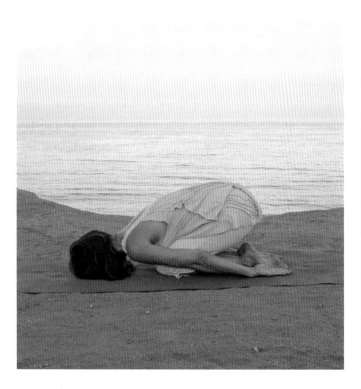 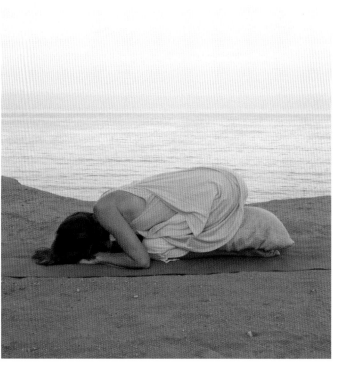

The Little-Known Sixth Rite

When Colonel Bradford returned from his discovery mission, he and Mr. Kelder taught classes on the Five Rites. Some time into this process, the Colonel revealed to Mr. Kelder that there is also a Sixth and lesser-known Rite -- a simple gesture, though it is unique in that is coupled with celibacy. This Rite was only to be performed when an individual felt complete with his or her sexual expressions. The exercise involves using one's breath to transmute sexual forces or energy upward to the other glands in the body.

Many people who have heard of the potential benefit of celibacy have simply abstained from sexual expressions or attempted to suppress their desires. It is completely different to draw or direct your sexual energy upward to other parts of the body. All other chakras in the body are affected by the first chakra, and it is believed to be life-altering to move this powerful energy up into the other glands and chakras.

For many years, a number of Eastern practices have advocated a slightly different approach: consciously choosing to abstain from *releasing* one's sexual energy while still sharing in the freedom of sexual activity. This enables a person to receive enjoyment of sexual activity *and* benefit from the vitality of this energy, instead of having to practice celibacy.

The Taoist belief is that there are a few powerful energies in the body. Along with chi, there is another energy that flows through the bodily fluids. The fluid that contains the greatest concentration of this energy is male semen. Taoist practices offer exercises for men, and women, to learn how to effectively redirect the powerful force of their sexual energy. They strongly believed that these practices were key to longevity, enhancing one's health and sexual experiences.

It is important for you to do what feels best in your body. Often, people will choose to be celibate for a specific period of time. Just as when we cleanse or fast from food, it can be an insightful time — one that enables us to see ourselves in a new light when we return to our everyday practices and lifestyles. A wide variety of books are available on these ancient Tantric sexual practices and Taoist exercises. This book's Sex and Longevity chapter offers a few simple exercises you can practice in fifteen minutes to enhance your sexual vitality and health.

For those interested in a celibate practice, the Sixth Rite follows, and this is *only to be practiced when you feel sexual desire and choose celibacy.*

- Standing upright with your knees soft, exhale completely as you bend forward placing your hands on your thighs. With the lungs empty, lift your body up.
- Place your hands on your hips and press them down toward the earth as you also pull your abdomen inward and lift your chest. Hold until you have to inhale.
- Inhale through the nostrils. As you exhale through the mouth relax your arms to your sides. Take several normal breaths.

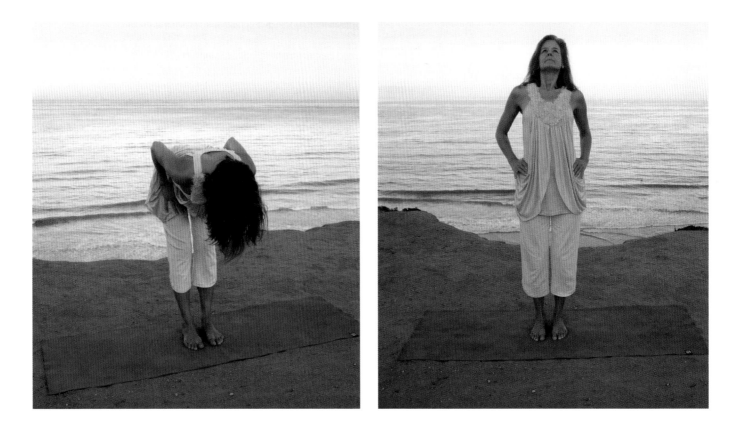

This would be one round of the Sixth Rite. Unlike the other Rites, *usually three repetitions* will enable the practitioner to feel a shift in their sexual desire. The Colonel referred to this Rite as what made the difference between a man or woman and a "superman or superwoman."

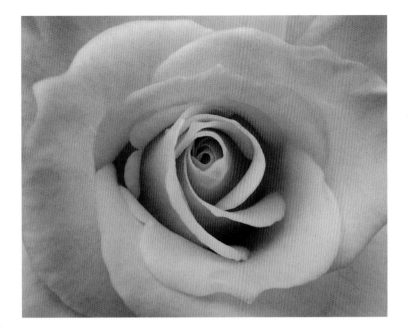

Enhancing the Five Rites

I have worked with the Five Rites throughout the last three decades and find them to be a gratifying beginning for strengthening my body. However, there are five important movements that I feel are valuable and necessary to add. The first is rotating or twisting the spine. The second is a lateral stretch of the spine. The third is developing balance. Especially as we age, balance is crucial to keeping us fall-proof. Fourth, is to stretch while on your belly. And, fifth, is an inversion.

I usually combine the Five Rites with yoga stretches that incorporate these additions. Consider adding poses from the following chapter whenever you work with the Rites for a more comprehensive experience.

You're never too old to become younger.

~ MAE WEST

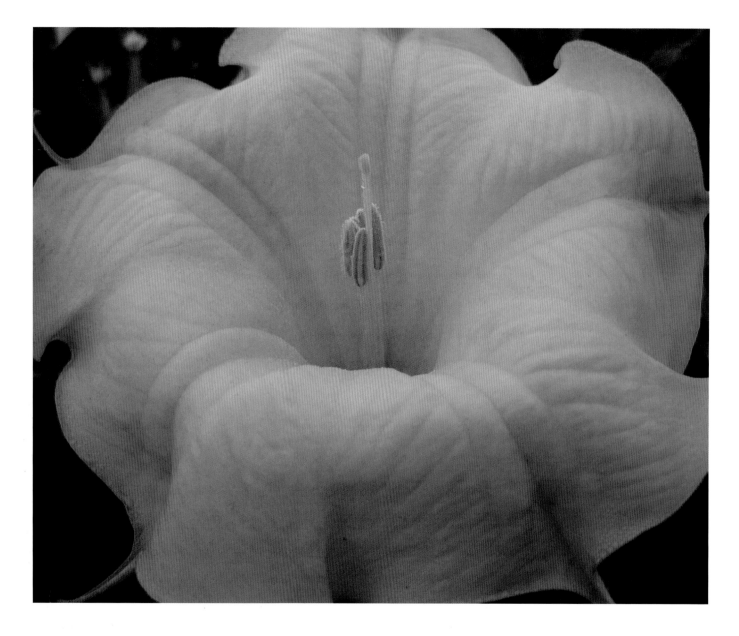

You have to leave the city of your comfort
and go into the wilderness of your intuition.
What you'll discover will be wonderful.
What you'll discover is yourself.

~ ALAN ALDA

Yoga:
enhancing your union with self

The meaning of yoga is union. The history of yoga dates back over 5,000 years, making it is the longest established system of self-improvement in the world. There are over a dozen recognized forms of yoga in the United States, offering nuances that enable students to explore a variety of styles.

Yoga works by clearing and strengthening our body, mind and spirit. Yoga is not a religion. It is a form of exercise that can enhance the quality of your life. You do not need to be religious or spiritual to practice the poses and receive the benefits. Practicing these stretches regularly is a preventive measure and helps maintain or improve the health of your spine, and your whole body.

While sampling many styles of yoga in my early practice, I encountered a few classes with dismay. I am deeply grateful that I did not let my first experiences of yoga discourage my quest to find a style that I liked, and I encourage you to experiment with different yogic styles to find the one that is a right fit for you. My training is primarily with Kripalu yoga, a Hatha-based yoga.

I have chosen a small and basic sampling of Hatha poses that enhance youthfulness by stretching your spine and body in all directions: forward and backward, laterally, into rotations and inverted. In combination or alternating with the Five Rites, with these poses you'll be able to create a comprehensive weekly workout. You should be able to do almost all of the poses in this chapter in a fifteen-minute practice.

Beyond stretching, balance is very important; it can help us to stay fall-proof by strengthening our focus and our ankles. I have included two balance poses and encourage you to explore others. Balancing poses highlight how naturally different one side of our body is from the other. Remember to be patient with *both* sides of your body.

The student volunteer models demonstrating the poses range in age from 55 to 90. Some of the models began practicing yoga in the past year. With creative modifications, age is not a factor.

Getting Started

All of the poses in this book can be done from sitting in a chair or lying on top of your bed. Some poses are demonstrated with a chair instead of standing. You may find it helpful to have a chair nearby for support in balancing, or to achieve a deeper stretch. You may also wish to stand against, or beside, a wall, especially if you are doing balance poses for the first time.

It is usually safest and easiest to perform yoga in your bare feet. If you are accustomed to always wearing shoes, experiment with practicing yoga without your shoes. It is safer, and healthier, to always keep your knees gently bent. Notice if you have a habit of "locking" your knees or elbows. Many people do this without realizing it. Chi practitioners feel that locking the elbows and knees weakens the body and sets joints up for potential risk of injury by interfering with the natural flow.

In the beginning, feel free to exaggerate the softening of your knees, almost as if you were going to squat or rest your tailbone upon the edge of a stool. Remember, yoga shouldn't hurt. If you have questions as to whether any of these poses are right for you, simplify the routine to the ones you can feel comfortable with. As you practice, you will develop more strength and confidence, enabling you to move into more challenging positions.

Every pose is demonstrated with modifications. Hold the poses only as long as you are comfortable. Pause in your poses so that you can focus more deeply on your breath, and develop your inner awareness. It is a wise choice to abbreviate the number of poses during your practice, especially in the beginning. Choose quality over quantity, and welcome a deeper connection and contentment in the poses you do perform.

Feel free to do the poses in any order that you are comfortable with, repeating as often as you like. It is best to have an empty belly and bladder while doing yoga. Plan to eat large meals at least an hour before practicing yoga. Lighter meals require less digestion time. You may also wish to experiment with playing soft music. Whenever possible, practice your stretches outside in fresh air.

Yoga is 90% about your breathing and 10% about stretching. When I first heard that in my training course, I assumed the instructor had mistakenly juxtaposed her words. As my practice has evolved, I've come to deeply appreciate the accuracy of this statement and the importance of our breath. The more you master your breathing, the more you embody the central benefit of yoga.

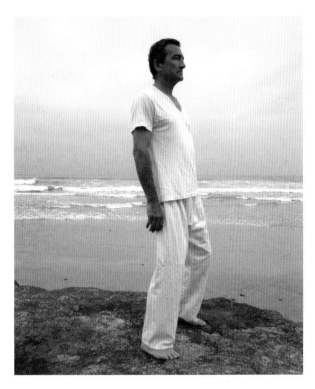

Model: *Tony Matarrese, 57 years young.*

Early practitioners knew that by placing their bodies in different positions, they could more efficiently oxygenate their blood, and strengthen, energize and heal their whole body. Kripalu yoga advocates holding poses or stretches as long as we are comfortable; this allows our *prana* (breath and life force) to access greater depths in our bodies.

There are contraindications for yoga poses, and if you question whether yoga is appropriate for you, please consult your physician. In general, if you choose to stand, your body will be working more. If you have a heart condition, you may wish to start off sitting or lying down on your bed. If you have high blood pressure, limit the amount of time you hold your arms up overhead. It can also be helpful to create a long pause in between your stretches. Listen to your body.

You will need a yoga strap for the first warm-ups. A tie or scarf will work equally well. For further information on yoga straps please consult my website, *www.naomicall.com.*

Warming Up

HIP AND LEG OPENERS

- Begin by lying down on your back, either on your bed or on the ground. Take a strap into one or both of your hands and place it around the ball of your right foot. Stretch your right leg up toward the sky.
- As you exhale, lower your leg toward the ground on your right side. Turn your head to the left.
- Inhale, and lift your leg up above your body. Bring your head back to center.
- Exhale, and lower your leg to your left side. Look to your right. Your hip will roll up, generating a deeper rotation. Look away from the direction you are moving your leg for a deeper twist.

Repeat as desired.

- Continue by circling your right leg in as large of a circle as possible. Cross over your body, so that your hip can roll up off of the bed or mat. Repeat as desired, and then circle in the opposite direction.
- Repeat the stretches on your left leg. Remember to inhale as you lift, and exhale as you release. Feel free to stretch your leg straight up toward the sky, or over your head. Pause, breathe and release.

MODIFICATIONS: Keep your knees gently soft and feel free to have pillows under your knees or around your hips for support.

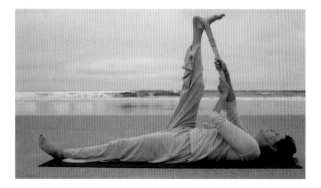 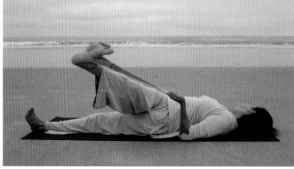

Model: *Jan O'Hara, 60 years young.*

Shoulder and Upper Body Openers

These stretches can be done sitting in a chair, or standing. From sitting, step your knees as wide as you can to create a strong foundation. If you are standing, step your feet as far apart.

- Take hold of your strap near the ends, you'll want as much length as possible. Inhale, and lift your arms as high as possible. This may be to chest or shoulder height. Honor your body, knowing you can work up higher as your body is able.
- Exhale, as you stretch your upper body and arms down to the right toward the ground. Look toward the sky.
- Inhale your arms back up.
- Exhale and stretch down to your left.

Repeat as desired, striving to stretch or breathe a little deeper each time.

MODIFICATION: Feel free to sit on the edge of your bed or chair. Please remember to only lift your arms as high as you are comfortable with.

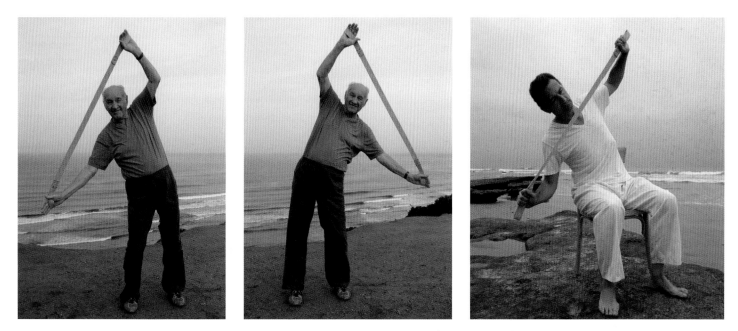

Model: *Cap Strawser, 89 youthful years.*

- Release your shoulders and strap down. Pause as needed. With your next inhalation, stretch your arms back up.
- Exhale as you twist to your right. Look back over your right shoulder.
- Inhale as you rotate your body forward.
- Exhale and stretch back to your left. Use your eyes to deepen the stretch by looking as far back as possible. Release your arms down.
- Repeat as desired.

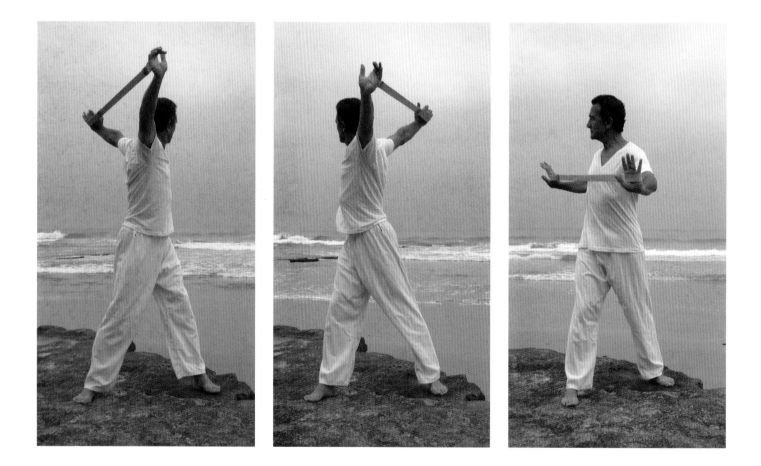

MODIFICATION: Feel free to modify by sitting on a chair or in bed for this stretch and the following one.

- Inhale and lift your arms up as far as you are comfortable, either to chest height, overhead or behind your back. Listen to your shoulders. Repeat as desired.
- Each time you lift, be aware of lifting your spine up off of your tailbone. Keep the space you are creating in your upper torso.
- As you release your arms down, do not compress the spine. Only your arms float down, so your body continues to feel taller and lighter. Remember to pause and consciously feel the space you are creating in your body.

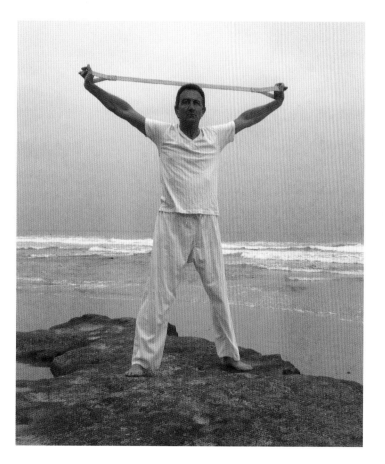

Key Poses for Longevity

Center: The Mountain Pose

The Mountain Pose is a tranquil and simple pose that often creates a foundation for other poses. You can do this pose sitting in bed, on a chair or standing.

- Bring your attention to your feet, and center your weight across your soles. Take a moment to gently rock forward and back on your soles.
- Explore bringing the sides of your big toes together so that your heels gently part. If you desire more stability, step your feet farther apart so that you are more firmly grounded.
- Stretch your toes as far apart as possible. Place your baby toes down on the ground, then your fourth toes, your middle toes, second toes, and finally your big toes. This is usually a challenge!

Many students did not believe this was possible until they saw it being done. It is easier if you look at your toes. It is a fascinating phenomenon that your fingers will often simultaneously attempt to do this!

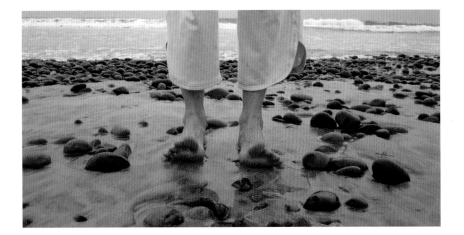

TIP: Walking on gently uneven surfaces in your bare feet is great way to energize and stimulate key acupressure points. Walking in the sand can also stretch and massage your feet. Find simple opportunities to strengthen and nourish your feet throughout your day. Choose shoes that have the smallest sole possible so that your feet are as close to the ground as possible. Find shoes that can conform to your feet.

- Soften your knees, as you tuck your tailbone and draw it toward the ground. Align your chin and the crown of your head to be parallel with the horizon.
- Inhale as you lift your arms away from the sides of your body, with your palms down. At shoulder height, rotate your palms toward the sky. Reach your arms as far up as comfortable. If possible, draw your palms together overhead and clasp your fingers. Pause.
- You may wish to close your eyes and envision a mountain. Feel your core strength. Breathe deeply into your belly and lift your spine up off of your waist standing even taller.
- Imagine the inner strength and stability of a mountain, even though the exterior is ever-changing, deep inside there is calm. Embrace what that feels like in your body. Regardless of external influences, sounds and energies, you are grounded and strong within yourself.
- To release, slowly lower your arms with your exhalation. At shoulder height, rotate your palms toward the earth. Maintain the lift you have created in your upper torso.

It is not the mountain we conquer, but ourselves.

~ SIR EDMUND HILLARY

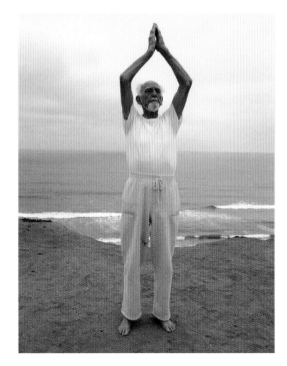

Model: *Vic Freudenberger, 91 youthful years.*

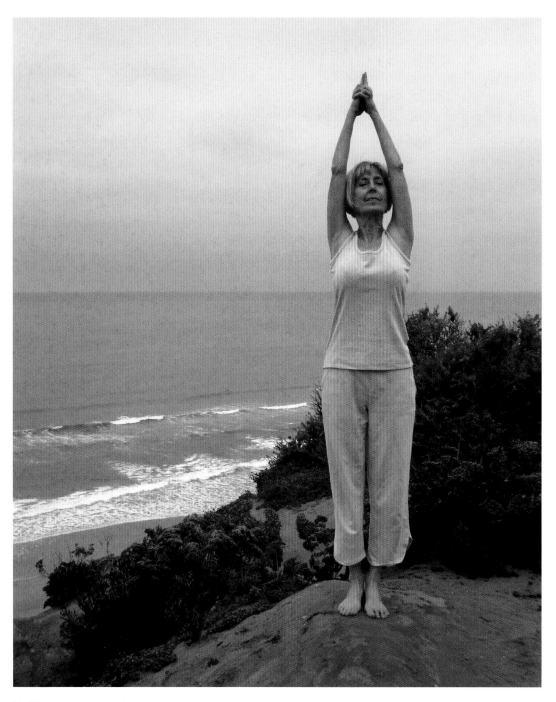

Model: *Donna Jacobsen, 65 youthful years.*

MODIFICATIONS: Feel free to sit, or have a chair beside you to hold onto for support, especially as you work with rocking your feet and stretching your toes. Draw your palms together at heart center and pause, or raise your arms as far as you can comfortably.

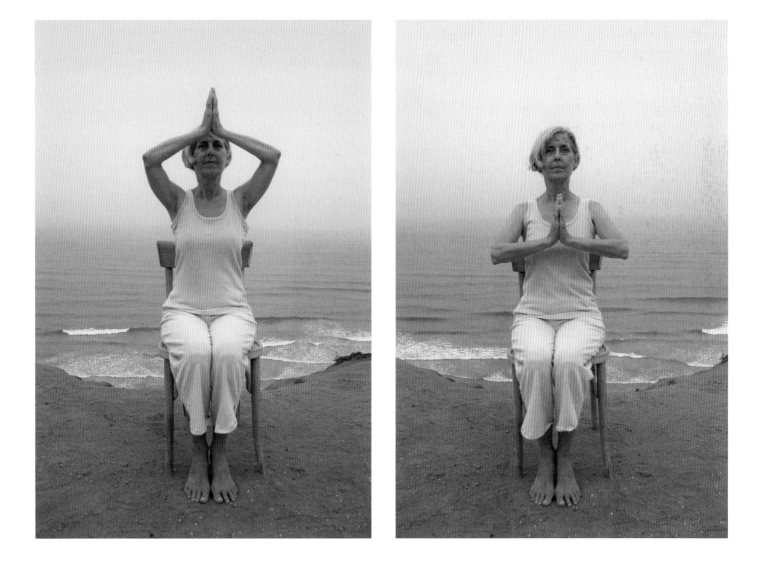

AFFIRMATION: *I am strong in my body, mind and spirit. I remain strong in the face of changes or challenges around me.*

Lateral Stretch: The Half Moon

I am drawn to all poses that relate to the moon. Many current styles of yoga emphasize the sun salutation, which is a more masculine flow of poses. I feel it is vitally important for women and men to honor and bring balance to their practice and lives by honoring their feminine wisdom and energy. If you would like to learn more about Moon Yoga, please visit *www.naomicall.com*.

- Bring your attention to your feet, and position your feet as wide as you need to create a stable foundation. Inhale your arms up into the Mountain Pose.
- Exhale, as you lengthen out toward your right. Strive to keep your upper shoulder rotated back. Pause.

Imagine that your body is in between two panes of glass. To keep from collapsing your right rib cage, press the heel of your right hand up into the heel of your left hand. This will keep your right side also equally stretching.

Forget not that the earth likes to feel your bare feet and the winds long to play with your hair.

~ KAHIL GIBRAN

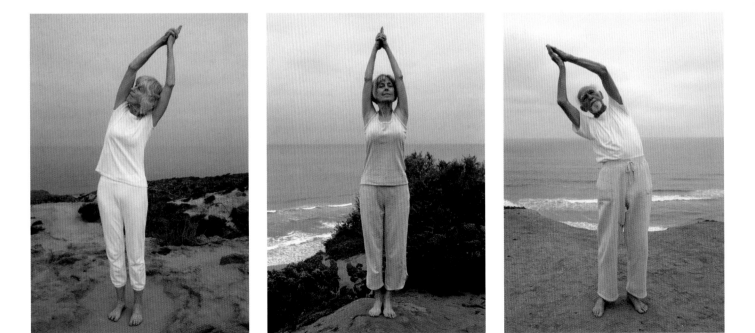

Model: *Julia Burgess-Perrot, 74 years young.*

- Inhale, and lengthen your body back to center in Mountain pose.
- Exhale as you lengthen toward the opposite side. Pause.
- Release on an inhalation bringing your arms back above your head. Release by floating your arms down to your sides.

MODIFICATION: Inhale and lift your arms to heart center instead of over your shoulders. As you stretch to each side, bring your attention to the crown of your head and imagine your body lengthening up as you also lengthen out.

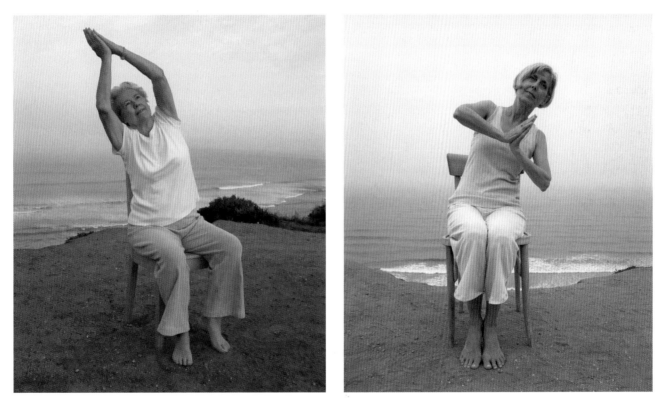

Model: *Pat Miller, 77 youthful years.*

AFFIRMATION: *I can effortlessly reach into new places in new ways. I have, or will be given, the tools I need for new beginnings.*

Balance: The Tree

The Tree is a favorite balancing pose for many people. It is simple enough that it can be modified for almost every body. Simply being close to a stable object, a wall or an actual tree, can provide a sense of security and stabilize your body.

- Take a few moments to bring your attention to the soles of your feet. Gently rock toward your toes and then sink back into your heels. Repeat a few times, or practice lifting your toes off of the ground and then placing them back down one at a time.
- Find a non-moving focal point in front of you and fix your gaze on it.

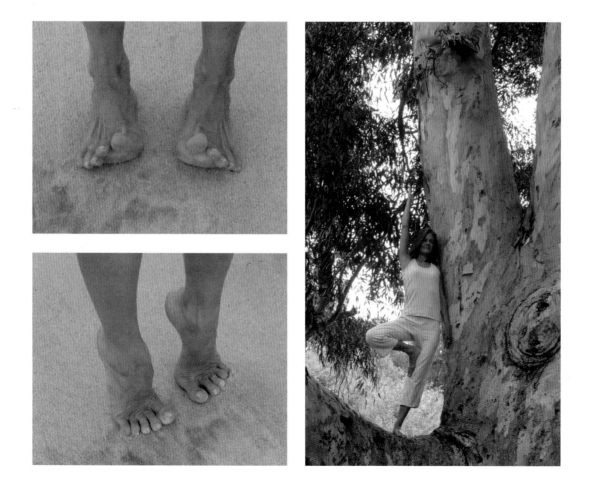

Sometimes our fate resembles a fruit tree in winter. Who would think that those branches would turn green again and blossom, but we hope it, we know it.

~ GOETHE

- Once your feet feel grounded, inhale as you lift your right foot. Take a moment to flex and circle your ankle and stretch your toes. Plant your foot either on the top of your left foot or somewhere against your left leg. Feel free to use your free hand to position your foot. Avoid placing any pressure on or behind the kneecap.
- Explore stretching your arms out to your side or overhead.
- Notice if you can take a deep breath. If you can't, modify or simplify your pose. Hold as long as you are comfortable.

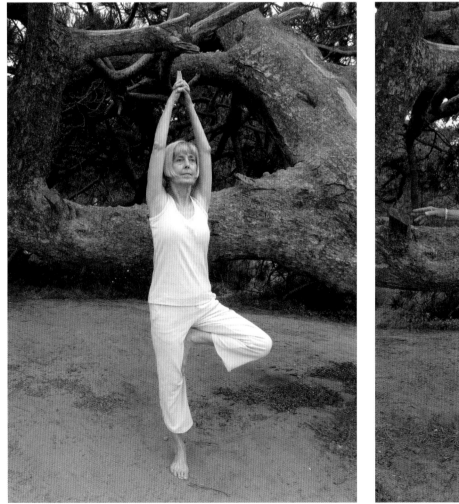

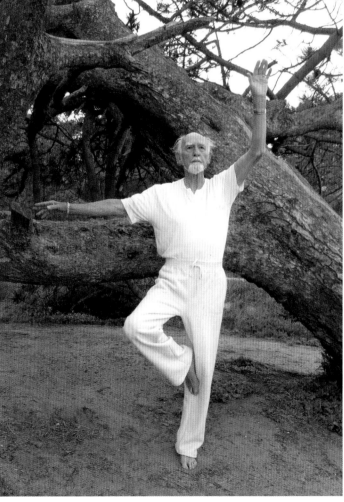

MODIFICATIONS: Bring your hands together at your heart center, or keep one hand on your chair or against the wall. Even a finger touching the wall or nearby tree can be helpful. You can also modify by using your hand to hold your foot up.

This pose can also be done sitting as a strengthening pose. Simply lift and hold your leg up or rest it on your other foot or leg. Breathe your arms up to your heart or overhead.

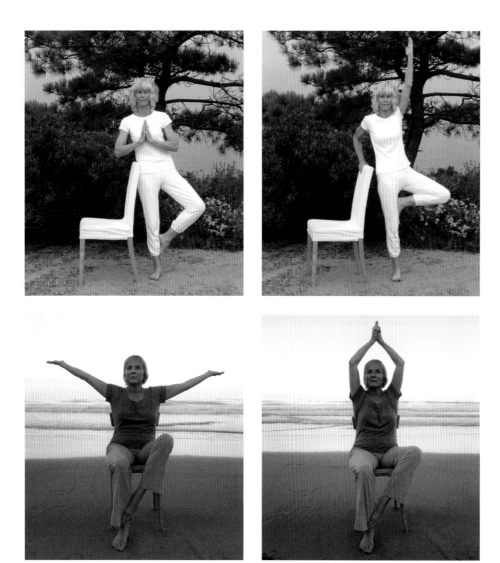

Model, bottom row: *Mary Hansom, 69 years young.*

As a wonderful hip opener, experiment with performing the *reclining* tree on your mat or on your bed. Feel free to place a pillow under your knee for additional support.

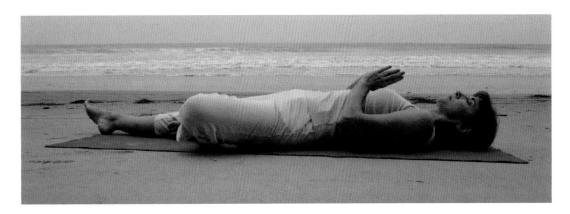

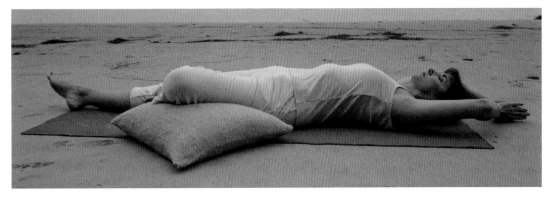

If balancing comes easily, bring in fluid movement to further develop your balance. Float one or both arms up and down, or softly bow forward and then back up. Focus on opening your hips by drawing back your knee that is lifted. Watch the tendency to hug the ears with the shoulders, and soften your shoulders down.

AFFIRMATION: *I am rooted and grounded. I am strong and in my heart and know what is best for me. I trust my inner guidance and connection with the earth.*

Model: *Marla Daigh,*
56 years young.

Counterbalance: The Balancing Half Moon

The Balancing Half Moon pose is one of the more challenging poses, though it can be modified. A chair, wall, or nearby tree will be helpful! You may wish to consider staying with practicing the Tree for a while as you build confidence and stability.

If using a wall, you'll be able to get more of a hip opening stretch. I encourage you to practice this pose with solid support. A wall will greatly enhance your ability to open your hips.

- Begin by standing close to a wall or tree. Step your feet farther than hip-width apart. Rotate your left foot to be parallel to the wall or tree.
- Gently float your right leg up from the ground. If possible, also allow your right arm to float upward. Feel free to hold the wall or tree for support. Your ultimate goal may be to bring your leg up parallel with the horizon.
- Take a deep breath and imagine pulling your right hip and shoulder up and back toward the wall. Hold for a few breaths if possible.
- This can be a very deep stretch, go easy and use your breath. Release.

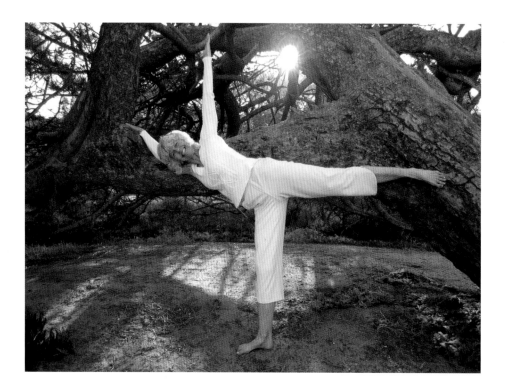

*The woman's mission is…
to express the feminine;
hers is not to preserve
a man-made world,
but to create a human
world by the infusion
of the feminine element
into all of its activities.*

~ MARGARET THATCHER

Repeat on the opposite side; remember to honor each side of your body. Be equally patient with both sides, expecting your performance to differ, versus pushing to be the same.

Model: *Julia, 76 years youthful, connecting with Torrey Pine.*

CHAIR MODIFICATION: Begin by stepping back to an arm's length from the chair. Slowly begin to lift your right leg while firmly holding onto the chair with both hands. You may want to slowly lift and lower you leg a few times. If it feels right, pause and hold your leg up. Breathe. If you are stable, experiment with floating your right hand up and off of the chair.

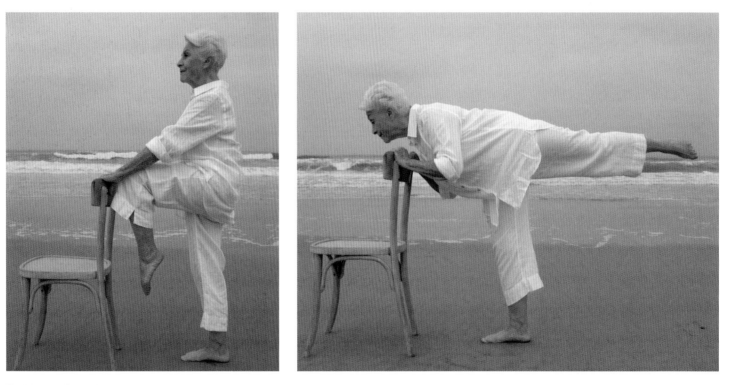

Model: *Brigit Clarke-Smith, 84 years young, demonstrates chair modifications.*

TIP: This is also a wonderful stretch to perform over the back of sofa. If you have a sofa that is not against a wall, or a railing in your home, these can be great props for helping to open your hips. If it is the right height, you may be able to rest your leg on the railing or sofa. The first two models are in their 70s and 80s who are doing this!

FLOOR OR BED MODIFICATION: You'll need either a chair or headboard within reach. Begin on your hands and knees. As you inhale, lift your right leg. Gently lift your right arm to the chair. Pause and breathe. You can release back down or experiment with reaching your right arm up toward the sky.

FOR A DEEPER STRETCH: Reach your upper arm back and take hold of your pant leg, ankle or foot. This can give you leverage to pull your hip up, and open. Hold, breathe and release. Repeat on the other side.

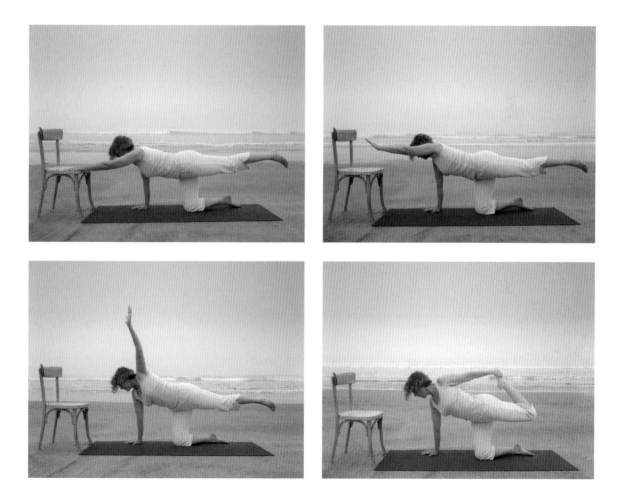

AFFIRMATION: *I am balanced. I honor my feminine and masculine, my light and dark, my soft and firm, my cool and warm, my sun and moon. It is my light that defines my shadows. I am grateful for both.*

Model: *Heather Martin*
57 youthful years.

101

Strength & Vision: The Warrior 1

This is a very strong pose. You may wish to prepare for this pose by first closing your eyes. Envision something that you are striving to achieve in life. See yourself doing or being that which you desire. *Feel it already being so.*

Or, if there is an affirmation that you are working with, repeat the affirmation, as you *feel it becoming so.* "I am youthful," for example. See your body, your hair and skin radiantly reflecting that which you desire. Don't suppress your desire or let your mind modify your ideal.

Gently re-open your eyes.

- Inhale, breathe your arms out to your sides, then if possible, up overhead. As you lift your arms, feel your upper torso lifting and expanding. Experiment with your hands separate and meeting.
- Exhale, and if needed, soften your shoulders down if they are lifted.
- Inhale and lift your right leg.
- As you exhale, step forward. Take a moment to firmly plant your feet. If you desire, you can drop your back heel by turning it in slightly. It is important to feel grounded and strong.
- Lift your spine up out of your waist. Feel yourself getting taller, creating space in your torso. If you wish, stretch into a gentle backbend. Imagine an invisible line from your tailbone up to the crown of your head. Like a puppet on a string, pull yourself up. Blossom your heart, possibly envisioning a beautiful multi-petaled flower.
- Pause and breathe. Repeat your affirmation or visualization as you lift your heart toward the sky. Float one or both of your arms out to your sides at shoulder height with your palms up. Breathe and feel the fullness of your life and of your image. Soften your arms down and step forward or back to release.

Repeat on the other side by stepping your left leg forward.

The indispensable first step to getting the things you want out of life is this: decide what you want.

~ BEN STEIN

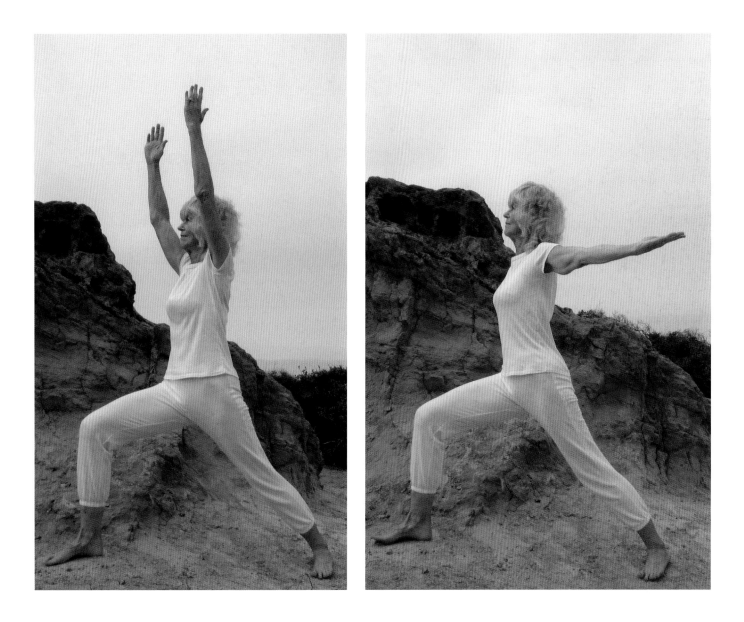

MODIFICATION: Simply draw your palms together at your heart instead of overhead. Or, keep one hand touching the back of a chair.

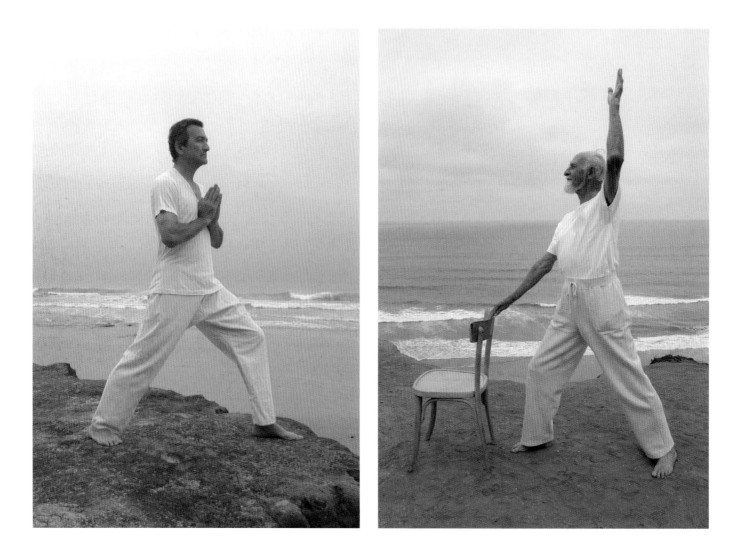

MODIFICATIONS: Have a chair nearby that you can step toward for support. Consider stepping forward with your arms down, either by your side or holding onto the chair for support. After stepping forward, and grounding your lower torso, then breathe one or both of your arms either to your heart or overhead. Create your pose from the ground up to be more stable.

If done sitting, position your body on the edge of your chair or corner of your bed, step your right leg back into a modified lunge. Breathe your arms up to your heart, out to shoulder height or up overhead. Feel your heart opening and your spine lengthening and lifting. Repeat with the other side.

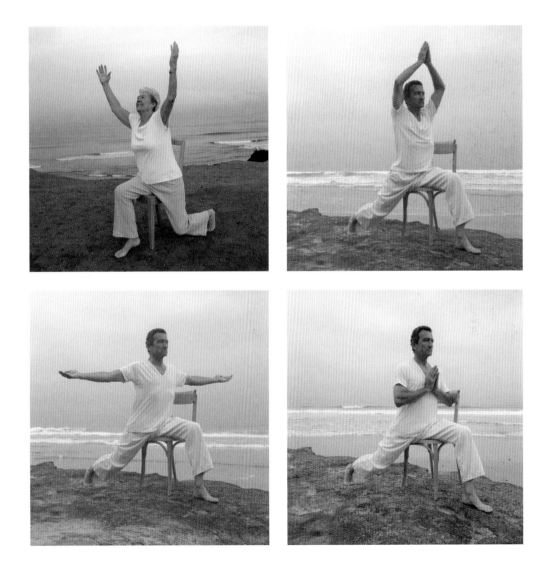

AFFIRMATION: *I can do anything. I step with confidence toward my dreams.*

Energize: Yoga Mudra

Yoga Mudra is known as the symbol of yoga and is one of my top-five favorite poses. This pose is a fabulous stretch to help counter everyday activities.

- From standing, position your feet farther than hip-width apart so that you have a strong foundation. Keep your knees soft, remembering not to lock them.
- Inhale, and float your arms up to shoulder height in front of your body and then around toward your back. Squeeze your shoulder blades together and feel the opening of your chest. Blossom and offer your heart toward the heavens.
- If possible, clasp your hands together. Pause as you press your knuckles toward the earth, deepening your stretch.
- Lengthen and hinge your upper torso forward. Come as far forward as you are comfortable with, pause, and take a deep breath.
- As you inhale, lift your arms up off of your torso, or simply imagine your hands to be floating up toward the sky.
- When you are ready to release, use your inhalation to help bring your body upright. Keep your hands clasped and imagine that there is a hook under your hands helping to lift your torso back up.
- Once upright, gently release your hands and allow the arms to float forward, and down. Often people experience a surge of energy upon releasing their hands.

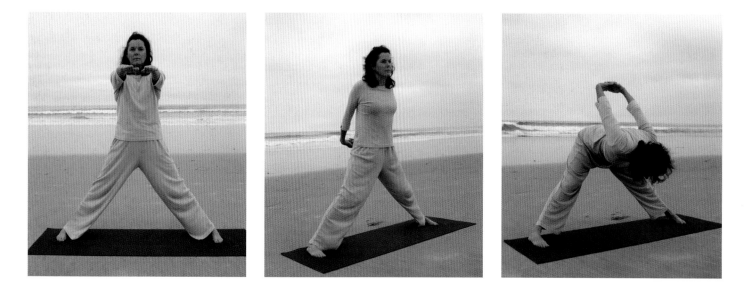

MODIFICATIONS: From standing, consider using a strap instead of clasping your hands together. Hinge forward as desired.

From sitting in an armless chair or stool: Step your knees apart to create a strong foundation. Inhale your arms behind your body. Modify as needed to achieve the deepest stretch. You may find it helpful to use the chair as leverage to draw your shoulder blades back and together. Bend as far forward as possible. Use your inhalation to bring your body upright.

*Let us not look
back in anger
or forward in fear,
but around
in awareness.*

~JAMES THURBER

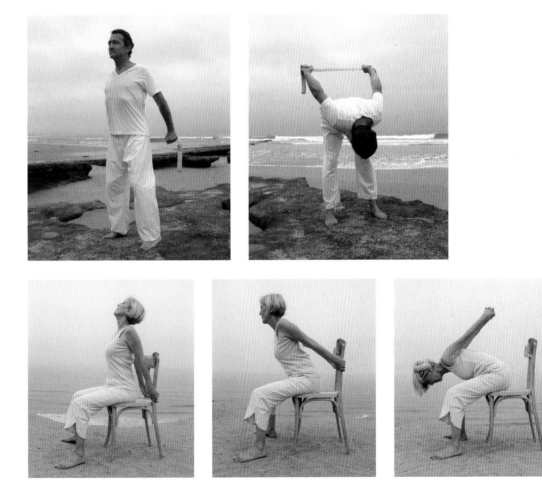

AFFIRMATION: *I delight in life. I love seeing new things in new ways.
I give thanks for all of life.*

Rotate: The Spinal Twist

Conscious rotations are fundamental to the health of the spine. Begin by sitting either on your mat, on a chair or on your bed. Take a moment to press your sit bones down as you lift your spine up off of your tailbone. Feel your body becoming taller. Twists originate in the base of your spine, not your shoulders.

- From sitting on the ground or a bed, lengthen your right leg out and press out through your right heel.
- Bend your left knee bringing your left sole to the ground or bed.
- Breathe in as you raise your left arm up to shoulder height. Fix your gaze upon your left middle finger as you slowly draw your left arm around behind your body.
- Midway, wrap your right arm around your left knee or press your right arm against the leg for leverage.
- Reach your left arm as far back as possible before releasing your arm down and placing your left palm on the ground or bed.
- Press your palm down as you again lift your spine up out of your waist and rotate further. Keep extending your stretch with your gaze.

Release and repeat on the other side. You'll be lengthening your left leg as you bend your right knee. Your right arm will float up and back behind your body. Wrap or press your left arm around your right knee for leverage.

TIP: The mind can get confused in a twist! It's easier if you remember that the arm that is *opposite* the extended leg is the arm that you draw behind your body.

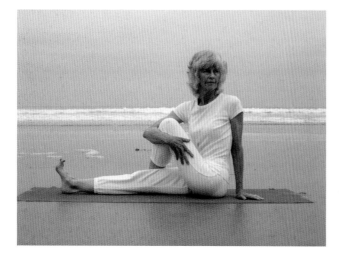
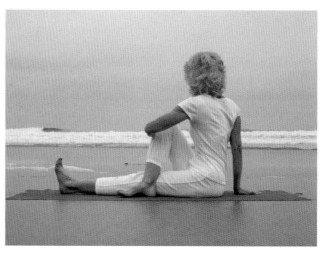

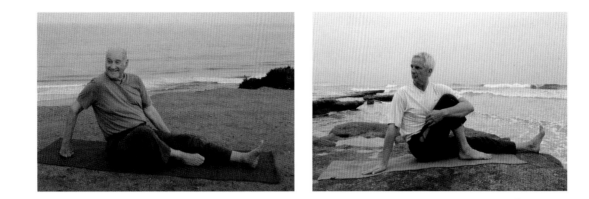

Model: *On the Left,
Harry Tracy, 57 years young.*

*We can never obtain
peace in the outer
world until we make
peace with ourselves.*

– DALAI LAMA

MODIFICATION: From sitting in an *armless* chair: Turn your knees all the way to your right side. With both feet on the ground, stretch your arms around to your right. Use the chair in any way that feels right to gain more leverage to rotate your body. Use your gaze to continue and accentuate your stretch. Continue lifting your spine and feel yourself being taller right up through the crown of your head. With each breath, notice if you can rotate further.

This is an easy stretch to incorporate into your workday and especially helpful if you have extended hours of sitting. Close your eyes for a moment and breathe. As you hold, notice if you can stretch any further.

TIP: If you are working on clearing feelings or thoughts from your past, twists can be very powerful poses. You may choose to have a gentle awareness of that which you are letting go while in your pose. As you take a breath and begin to unwind and release your body, affirm that you are also releasing your past. Specifics aren't needed; simply your intention will be enough.

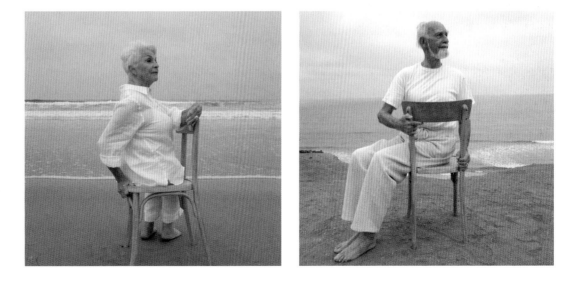

AFFIRMATION: *I appreciate the front and the back of every aspect of my life.*

The Table

This simple pose can be the starting point for the Cat & Dog and Pigeon poses.

- Begin by placing your knees under your hipbones, and wrists under your shoulders.
- Keep your elbows gently soft. Softly gaze toward the earth as you release the creases in the back of the neck.

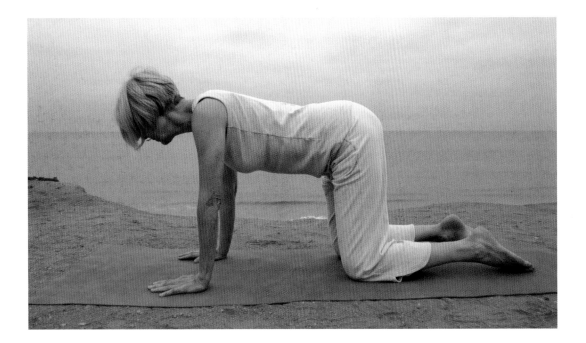

Spinal Stretch: The Cat & Dog

Cat & Dog Pose is an energizing warm-up for your spine and preparation for the Pigeon.

- Begin in Table Pose.
- As you inhale, lift your tailbone and the crown of your head toward the sky.
- Exhale as you tuck your tailbone and chin.
- Repeat as desired.

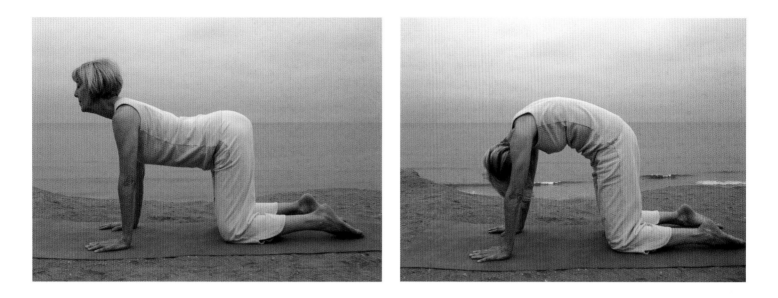

MODIFICATION: This can be done in a chair, or on your bed. As you inhale, simply lift your spine up as you squeeze your shoulder blades together. As you exhale, tuck your chin and softly round your spine and bend forward.

If sitting in a chair, you can experiment with using your chair as leverage. As you inhale up, grab hold of your chair to help pull back and open the upper torso even more. Feel free to bend as far forward as you like.

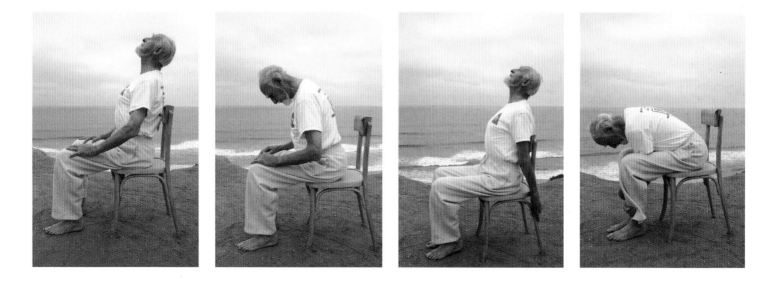

Hip Opener: The Pigeon

This pose is a favorite hip opener with most yoga practitioners. It can be performed on your bed or on the ground.

- Begin on all fours, in what is known as a Table pose, (see page 110).
- Draw your right knee forward, between your hands.
- Imagine your hips to be like headlights, equally shining forward. Lift your spine up, out of your waist, as you lengthen your body forward to the earth or bed. Soften as far over as possible. If your forehead is not touching the ground or your bed, feel free to use pillows, or stack your fists to rest your forehead on.

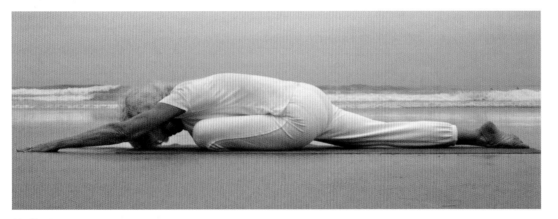

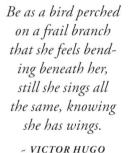

Be as a bird perched on a frail branch that she feels bending beneath her, still she sings all the same, knowing she has wings.

~ *VICTOR HUGO*

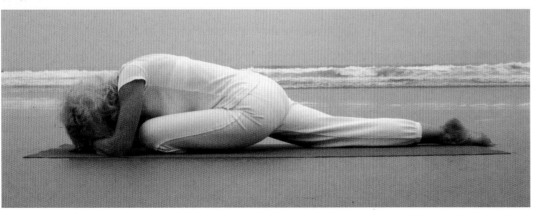

- Pause and breathe, feel your hips opening. Hold as long as you desire.
- On an inhalation, press your palms to the earth as you bring your body upright. Feel free to pause with your hands on your mat, bed or on your thighs. As you breathe, continue to lift your spine up. Have a sense of blossoming and opening your heart, your throat and the crown of your head. Stretch as far back as you desire.
- Release, and repeat on the other side.

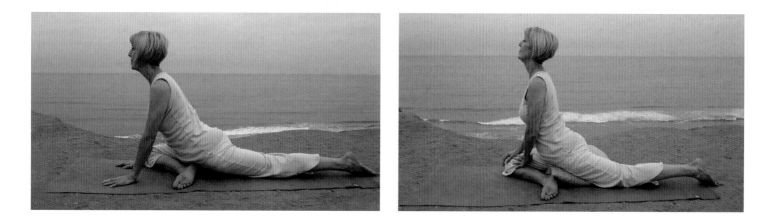

MODIFICATION: Place a pillow(s) or rolled blanket under your buttock for support. You may also wish to have a pillow(s) for under your forehead or simply stack your fists or forearms.

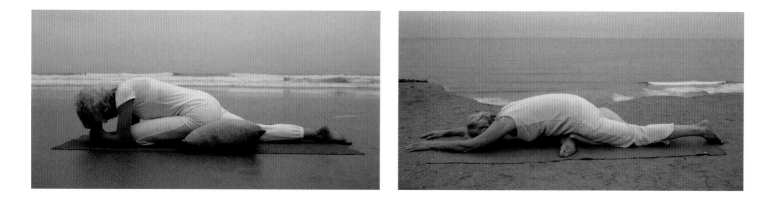

AFFIRMATION: *I surrender, open to receive, connect and soar into my dreams.*

Nourish: The Sphinx or Cobra

There are a number of poses done with your belly on the ground, which are equally wonderful for nourishing and toning all of your organs. A good beginning is the Sphinx, possibly followed by stretching into the Cobra.

- Begin by simply resting on your belly, feeling your breath.
- As you inhale, press your belly toward the earth. As you exhale, imagine peeling your navel up off of your mat or bed. Repeat a few times.
- If you are not outside, visualize being outside lying in a favorite place. Imagine the warm sand, or the feeling of the earth's energy and support. Relax completely into that support.
- Bring your forearms up toward your head on your mat with your palms down. Keep your elbows tucked in, resting your forehead on your mat or your bed. Press your pelvic area down as you inhale and lift your chin and chest up. Have a sense of leading your pose from your sternum or breastbone.
- Press the crown of your head up toward the sky. Keep your shoulders soft, pressing them *down* toward the earth. Come up as far as your body wants and pause. Feel free to be fluid, and repeat as desired. Continue to use your breath to nourish your body.

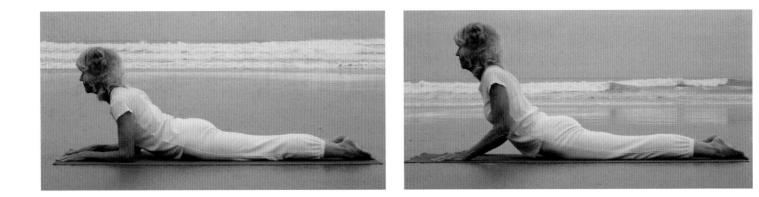

DEEPER STRETCH, THE COBRA: If you wish, bring your palms to your mat instead of the forearms. The Cobra Pose will enable you to lift higher. Press into your palms and inhale up. Again, your shoulders stay soft and press down toward the earth. Hold as desired. Release with an exhalation as you *lengthen* your body down. Imagine that you are placing your forehead onto the earth far beyond your mat.

MORE BELLY DOWN POSES: I feel all of these are very beneficial and encourage you to explore further. They are the Bow, Half Bow and Locust.

Harry demonstrates below a variety of other belly down poses that I feel are very beneficial if you wish to experiment further.

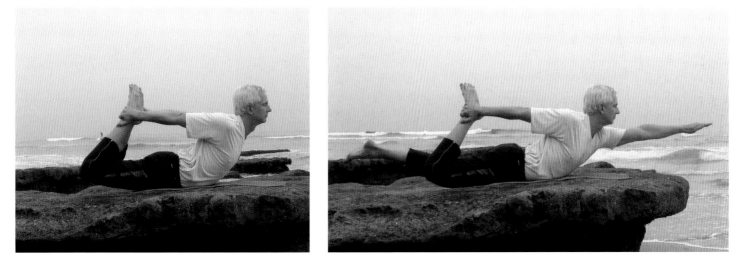

Gratitude bestows reverence, allowing us to encounter everyday epiphanies, those transcendent moments of awe that change forever how we experience life and the world.

– JOHN MILTON

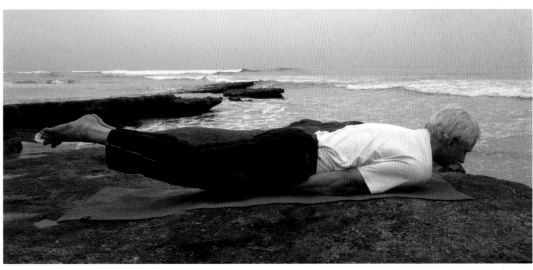

AFFIRMATION: *I shed the skin of my past with honor and gratitude. I welcome new beginnings with greater strength and clarity.*

Restore: The Child

This is a restorative pose that can be modified to provide deep relaxation and healing. The child can be performed on the ground or on your bed. It's nice to do first thing in the morning on your bed and is a perfect counter stretch for any backbend or belly-down pose.

- Holding this pose can help lengthen your spine. There are numerous variations and props to support and accentuate the benefits and pleasure that you can receive.
- It is usually easiest to begin in the table pose, see page 110. As you exhale, allow your hips to soften toward your heels, gravity will help you surrender. Use as many pillows or rolled blankets as you need. Experiment with different heights and combinations until it feels perfect. Your arms may rest along the sides of your body, tucked in between your legs or lengthened overhead on your mat or bed. If you don't have a pillow for your head, you can also make fists with your hands and rest your forehead on your wrists.
- Hold and deeply breathe. As you inhale feel your belly pressing against your thighs.

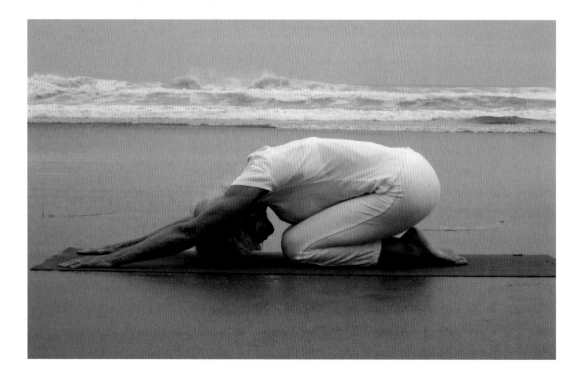

There is a garden in every childhood, an enchanted place where colors are brighter, the air softer, and the morning more fragrant than ever again.

– ELIZABETH LAWRENCE

TIP: For a rejuvenating abdominal massage, make loose fists and place your fists on your thighs before bending forward. Once you have hinged forward, experiment with gently rotating your wrists.

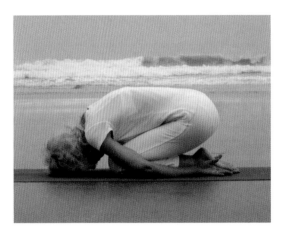

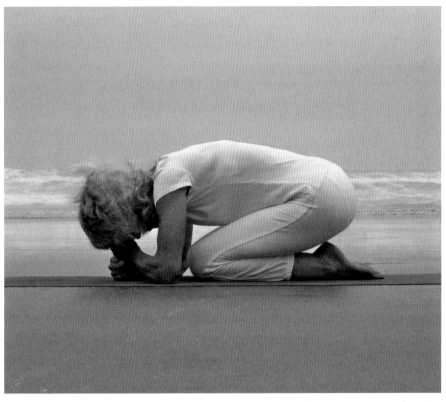

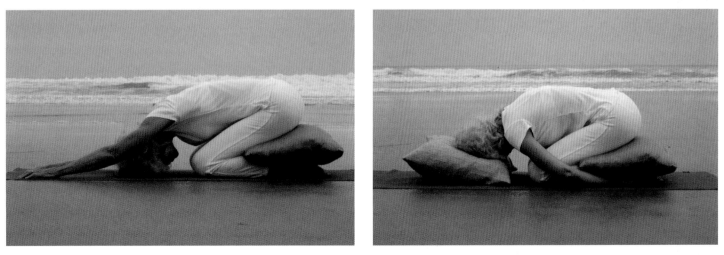

AFFIRMATION: *I am a shining spirit, safe and protected. I am blessed.*

Shift: The Single Knee-Down Twist

This pose can be done on the ground or on your bed. This is a highly beneficial pose that almost anyone can do. If you only have time to do one pose, this is often a good one. Taking time out of your day to pause and bring your body into a horizontal position can immediately begin to shift your focus and your energy.

- Have pillows or blankets available to support your body as you explore possible modifications. A strap can also be helpful in drawing your knee up.
- From a lying down position on your back, take a moment to breathe deeply as you lengthen your spine and body out. Feel the support of the earth under you.
- Inhale and draw your right knee toward your chest.
- Exhale as you stretch your knee toward or over your left leg. The right foot can stay to the right side of your left leg, or feel free to explore stretching your right leg completely over the left leg.
- Adjust your spine, shoulders and upper torso as needed so that you are able to luxuriate in this pose. Totally surrender and feel the support of gravity and the earth. Rotate your head to look toward the right. Pause and breathe. With each breath, feel your body letting go and opening a little further to receive.

Repeat on the other side, honoring the difference of your left and right sides. Remember to turn the head away from the direction your leg is moving.

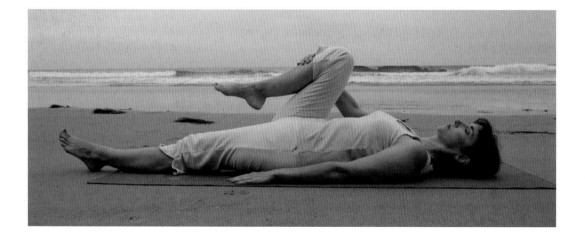

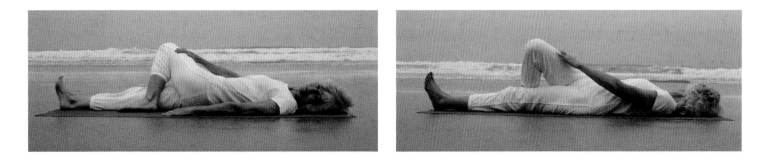

MODIFICATIONS: Support your bent knee with blankets or pillows. Consider using a strap to facilitate your stretch and support your leg. If you are unable to lie comfortably on your back, begin by lying on the right side of your body and move into your twist from the side instead.

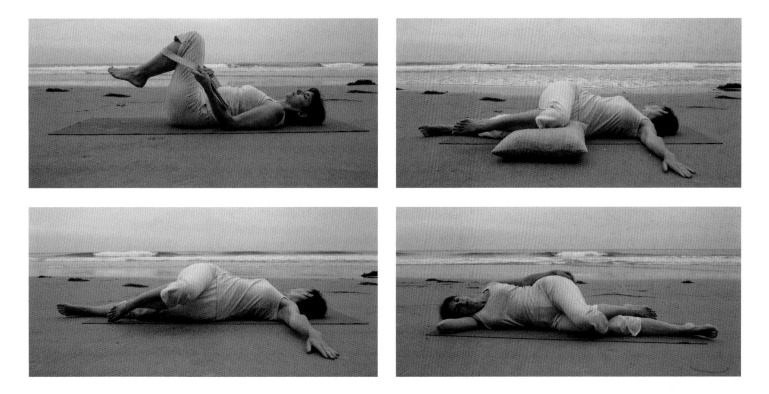

AFFIRMATION: *I am flexible. I open to seeing situations in a new light. I can flow with the energy around me.*

Inversion: Legs Up the Wall (or Tree)

Inversion poses are a key to longevity. Inversions can relieve pressure on the abdominal organs and the veins, stimulate the brain, increase circulation and enhance glandular and hormonal function, especially for the thyroid. As with most poses, there are simplified versions to adapt to just about every body. The most restorative variation is usually what is simply referred to as Legs Up the Wall. You can also place your legs against a headboard, a chair or a tree for added benefit of being connected with nature.

- Begin by lying down on your side, on your bed or the ground. Position your buttocks right up against the wall, a headboard, a chair or a tree. Feel free to put a rolled towel under your neck, or blanket under your spine or tailbone for cushioning.
- Walk your legs up the supporting surface as you rotate your upper torso in alignment with your legs. Ideally, the backs of your legs are fairly flush with your support surface. Adjust so that it feels wonderful. Many people find this so restorative that they stay for 15 minutes just in this pose!
- If you suffer from water retention, swelling, varicose veins or aching feet or legs, this is a heavenly pose. I have yet to meet someone who didn't like this.

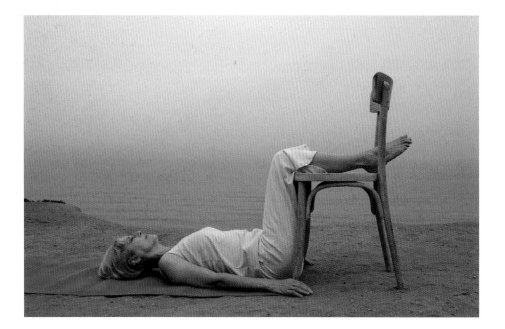

"Who am I, and where am I going? You are the answer to this question. You are here to ask the question, and to be the answer."

– REV. MICHAEL BECKWITH

Being upside down can open our minds and enable us to see life in a whole new way. If you want to change your mood or feel stuck or stressed, experiment with taking a break and putting your legs up. Consider adding an aromatherapy pillow over your eyes or some soothing music, and enjoy feeling "transported" to a different place.

NOTE: People with heart or eye conditions are cautioned to check with their doctor to confirm if inversions are best for you. It is usually best to abstain from inversions if you are menstruating.

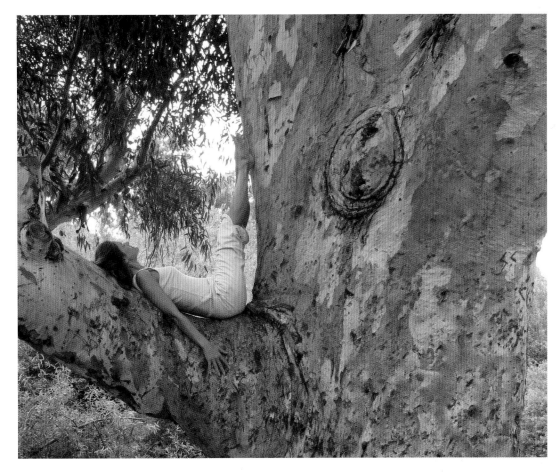

MODIFY FOR DEEPER STRETCH: Feel free to add cushions or stacked blankets at the base of the tree or wall to lift your tailbone up higher, creating more of a lift.

AFFIRMATION: *I love and appreciate seeing my life and the world in new ways.*

Smile: The Happy Baby

This pose often brings a sense of playfulness and a smile. Feel free to add this into your routine if you enjoy it. It can be very relaxing, and can be done on your bed or on the ground.

- Begin on your back. Draw your knees up to your chest in a pose that is known as a Reverse Child. Clasp your hands around your thighs, or over your shins.
- Feel free to pause and gently rock or circle your body.
- Separate your legs as you reach your arms between your legs, and your hands to your legs or feet. Allow your soles to float toward the sky, keeping your knees soft. Drop your legs apart as far as is comfortable for you.
- If you feel vulnerable in this pose, take a deep breath and notice your feelings. Close your eyes and move into your feelings with a deeper breath. Trust.

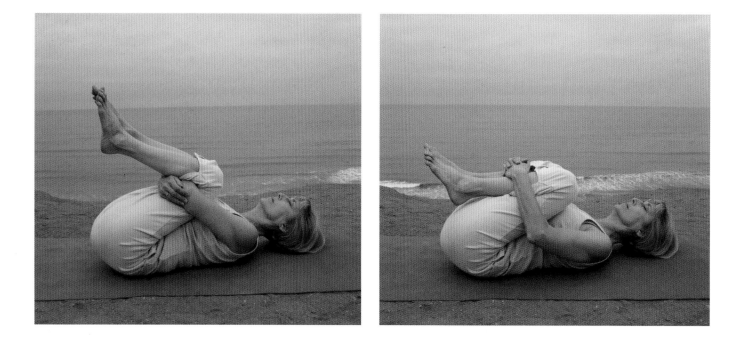

- Roll from side to side, possibly even rolling all the way to the side and then pushing off as you lift and roll to the other side.

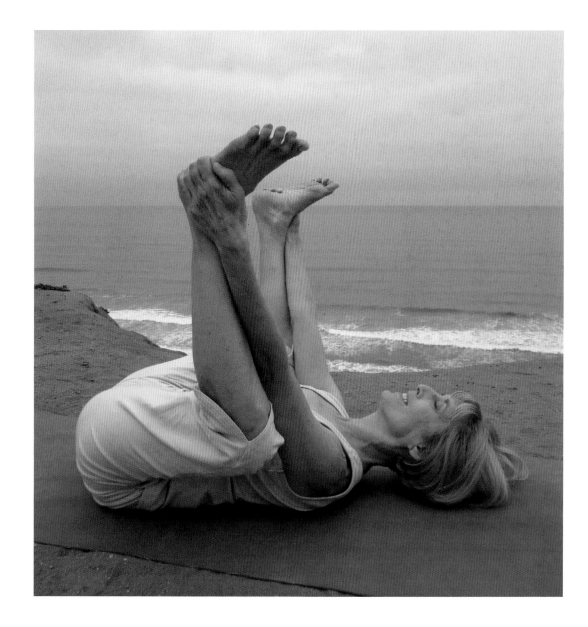

"He who laughs, lasts."

~MARY PETTIBONE
POOLE

Have fun!! Smile. Keep your attention on your breath or take a few moments to recall some of your favorite childhood moments, re-living in your mind's eye your child-like wonder and joy.

AFFIRMATION: *I am joy. I celebrate my bliss and my blessings!*

For flexible practitioners, there is also an ancient practice of "weaving" your toes together. Using your hands, wedge your toes in between each other. This is another way to deeply nourish all of the meridians in your toes at the same time. Once you are in this position, roll your body in a circular motion and feel your toes awakening. This is a good follow-up to your Do-In practice!

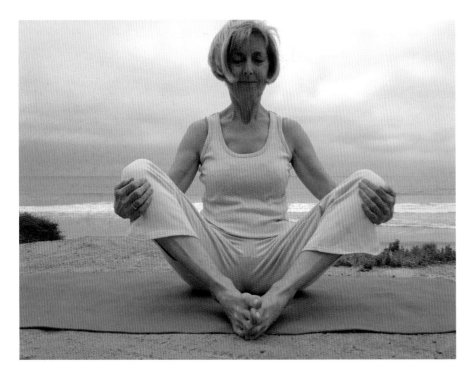

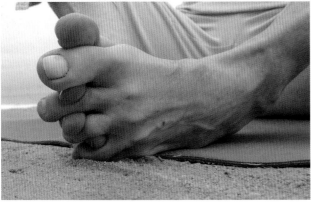

"The human foot
is a masterpiece
of engineering and
a work of art."

~ *LEONARDO DA VINCI*

When we practice yoga, we can see the world in a fresh light, from a view previously unimaginable. As we stretch to new heights, our trust deepens, and we find our union. Our body, mind and soul are one, present in this unrepeatable moment.

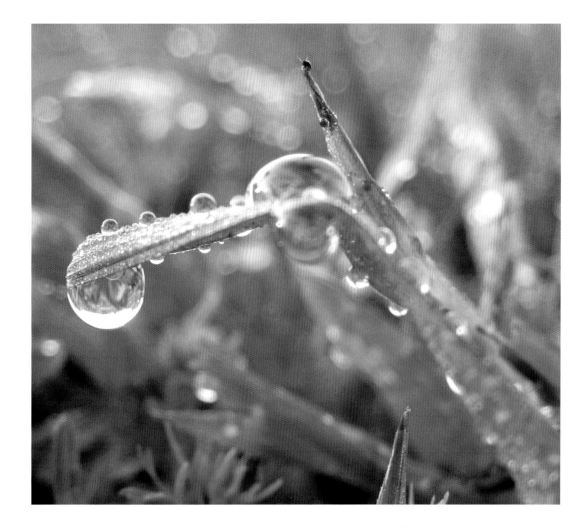

"Things are not as they appear,
nor are they otherwise."

~ LAKOTA WISDOM

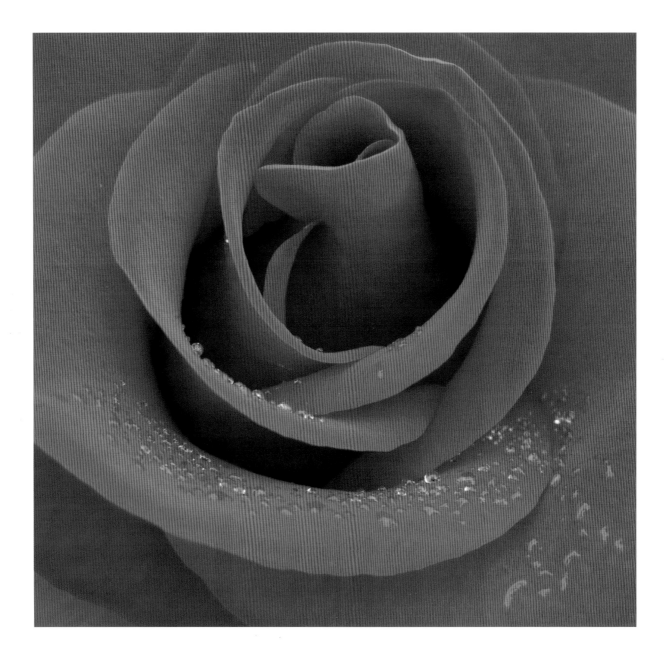

Sex is an emotion in motion.

~ *MAE WEST*

Sex and Longevity: keeping your fire burning

It Starts in the Glands

Ancient Taoists recognized that the health of our sexual glands is fundamental to the well-being and function of our body, mind and spirit. Each gland in your body is dependent upon the other glands to receive the energy and fluid it needs to perform its task. The sexual glands form the foundation of our glandular system. There are seven major sexual, or endocrine glands — glands that produce hormones — which are as follows:

GONADS – In men, they are the prostate and testes. In women, they are the ovaries, uterus and mammary glands or breasts. Their functions are hormone secretion and guiding sexual energy and responsiveness.

ADRENAL GLANDS – Located just above the kidneys, they support the kidneys in regulating the effects of stress on the body.

PANCREAS – Behind the stomach, deep in the body, the pancreas helps to regulate digestion and blood sugar levels.

THYMUS – Positioned behind the sternum, this gland oversees the heart, lungs and bones.

THYROID – This gland in the neck stimulates and synchronizes all metabolic cellular functions. All tissues and vital anti-aging hormones are affected by its functioning.

PITUITARY – Located just below the brain, this gland controls the mind, intellect and thought processes. Often called the "master gland."

PINEAL – Set deep inside of the brain, this gland affects all other glands and is believed to deepen one's connection to spirit or higher knowing and intuition.

Endocrine glands release over 20 hormones directly into the bloodstream where they can be transported to cells in other parts of the body. When any one of these glands is depleted, the functioning of another is compromised.

The Chinese believed that if any of the first six glands were not performing fluidly, their spiritual awareness and ability to connect to God or Divine awareness would be limited. Many energy practitioners engage in a number of exercises to strengthen their sexual energy, knowing that this center is the foundation of all other centers in their body. The Taoists liken the sexual center to a stove that, when properly filled with energy, will alight with fire that will then serve to warm, feed and stimulate the whole house or body. As always, it is important to not overdo, and to maintain the proper balance.

Taoist "Ching"-Inspired Exercises

Taoists refer to sexual energy as "ching." The male sexual essence or ching can release 200 to 500 million sperm in a single ejaculation. The production of this fluid can consume up to one third of a man's daily energy output. Therefore, Taoists were conservative both about releasing this fluid and replenishing it, so not to age or diminish their forces prematurely.

Following are contemporary Western exercises and ancient Taoist energy practices that enhance sexual energy. There are versions for men and women.

TAOIST DEER EXERCISE

It is known that by exercising the anal muscles and rectum that the sexual glands are stimulated. The Chinese believe that the simple action of a deer continually flicking its tail stimulates its sexual glands. This energy then rises into the deer's glandular system and ultimately into its antlers. For centuries, the horns of a deer have been esteemed for their potent medicinal value.

The conscious use of sexual energy is widely recognized as a key to longevity. The following exercise helps to replenish one's sexual energy that is lost in the act of sexual activity. Even if you are not sexually active this is an important exercise.

If you have a sense of having drained your sexual energy, you may wish to couple the exercise with visualization as you practice. See your breath as light, and feel yourself becoming more radiant. Remember that your thoughts are a reality. Connect into your roots. Envision this light to be nourishing every cell of your body.

As we get older, the anal muscles and rectum can loosen and become weakened. The Deer exercise strengthens theses muscles and the control of the bowels. Along with the numerous physical benefits, including increased fertility, the clarity and functioning of our mind and our spirit is greatly enhanced.

THE DEER EXERCISE FOR MEN

During the deer exercise, men engage the sphincter muscle, which also benefits the prostrate. This can help to prevent and even reverse diseases associated with the prostate including cancer, enlargement, hemorrhoids, weakness and dysfunction.

This exercise can be performed from either standing or lying down, and ideally touching your hands to your skin.

- Begin by rubbing your hands together to bring more energy into your palms. With your right hand, gently cup your entire scrotum. Feel the warmth of your palm.
- Place your left hand on your abdominal area approximately one inch below your navel. Rotate your hand in a clockwise circle with enough gentle pressure that it warms your pubis area.

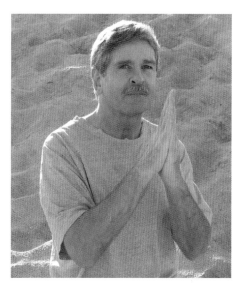 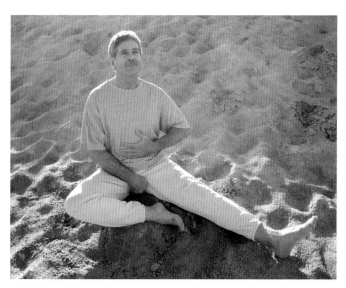

This exercise is ideally performed 81 times, meaning that you rotate your hand 81 circles. The Taoist have high regard for the sacredness in numbers and believe that every number has significance. The numbers 8 and 1 add up to a 9. This number has the highest possible Yang energy. You may wish to start simply with any multiple of nine. Repeat the same number on the other side.

- Begin by again rubbing your hands together to re-warm and energize. Place your left palm over your scrotum and now rotate your right hand over the pubic area.
- For the second part of this exercise, squeeze the anal muscle as tight as you can without creating stress. Hold as long as possible, release and repeat as desired.

Persistence will provide you with control of this muscle and the difference can usually be felt within a few weeks. Often a pleasant feeling is associated with this exercise as contraction of this muscle places pressure on the prostate gland. This energy will feel as though it is traveling up the spine, as it is being diverted to the pineal gland. When you have mastered squeezing this muscle, you can perform this exercise together with or independent of the first part of the deer exercise.

There are numerous benefits to strengthening the rectum and prostate, including the strengthening of nerve endings in the pubis and prostate that can facilitate healing impotence and premature ejaculation. Heightened pleasure is also often a result.

THE DEER EXERCISE FOR WOMEN

- Sit either on the floor or on your bed.
- If possible, bring the heel of one foot up to your groin, and press the heel firmly against the opening to your vagina and clitoris. If you cannot press your heel in, substitute with another object that can place pressure against your clitoris. A tennis ball works well. You may experience a pleasant stimulation.
- Rub your palms vigorously together warming them up. Place your hands on your breasts and feel the warmth on your skin. Begin to circle your hands in an outward gesture for 36 repetitions. Modify as needed so as to not create stress or overtire your arms. For example you may start with fewer and work your way up to 36 repetitions.

When you move your arms in an outward movement you are dispersing energy away from your breasts. This helps to prevent energy from stagnating and forming lumps or cancer in the breasts. This exercise can also be reversed so that you are drawing energy into the breasts to help nourish the tissue, and in effect, enlarge the breasts.

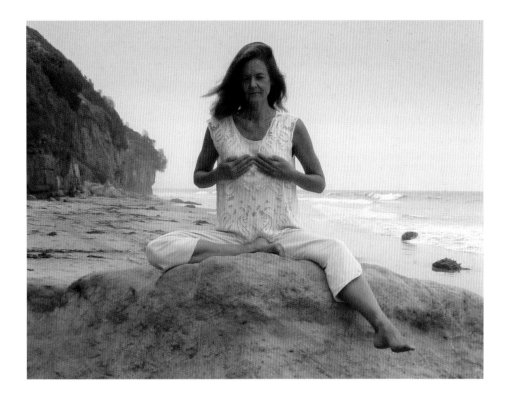

Bring your undivided attention and clear intention to what you are doing. Be present, do not let your mind wander elsewhere. When you have completed rubbing your breasts, release your hands.

Bring your attention to the muscles of the rectum and pubococcygeus muscle (PC muscle), also known as the Kegel muscle, the muscle you would use to stop urination in mid-stream. Squeeze these muscles, creating a sense of closing off your vagina and anus. You may feel warmth or energy floating up your spine.

These exercises help to create youthfulness and beauty by strengthening your sexual organs and function. They also can remedy a host of physical ailments from vaginal disorders to menstruation difficulties. Please note that women are advised to *not* perform the deer exercise during menstruation or pregnancy.

In yogic meditation practices the control of these muscles are referred to as "locks." It is believed that by masterfully applying these locks, or squeezing these muscles, one gains the ability to raise their sexual energy, consequently strengthening their spiritual center. This will then enable a practitioner to reach new heights in their meditation practice.

PROPER SITTING PRACTICES

Both men and women can practice sitting with one heel, or a firm object, pressed against the scrotum or clitoris. The other leg can be lengthened out or also bent and folded toward the body in a tailor, or lotus position.

Taoists believe that sitting in this position helps to guard against the loss of energy through what they call the "gate of heaven." Whether you have engaged in an excess of sexual activity or abstained from sex, your sexual organs can weaken if you are not consciously building forces.

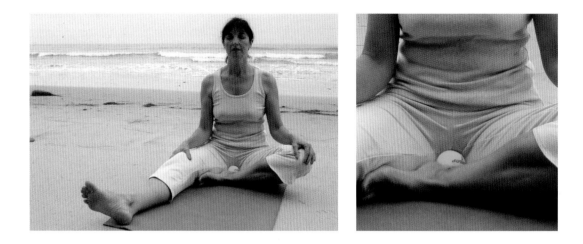

Kegel Exercises *(The "Stoplight Exercise") for Men & Women*

The following exercise is named after Dr. Arnold Kegel. The Kegel exercise consists of contracting and relaxing the muscles that form part of the pelvic floor (which some people refer to as the "Kegel muscles"). These exercises improve your muscle tone by strengthening the pubococcygeus muscle (PC muscle). Many women are prescribed these exercises when pregnant, as a tool for thwarting off urinary incontinence that arises most commonly after vaginal childbirth. Sadly, men are not usually informed as often about the benefits these exercises also hold for them.

Research has found that Kegel exercises can help with a number of conditions along with incontinence in both men and women. Many men report having stronger erections, restoring erectile weakness and eliminating premature ejaculations. Some men experience enhanced and multiple orgasms after strengthening their awareness and use of this muscle.

Model: *Marla Daigh, 56 years young.*

These exercises are simple to do, and the joy is that you can do them anywhere and at any time, without anyone ever knowing. Hence the nickname, "stoplight exercise." My midwife suggested doing one hundred Kegels a day in a series of repetitions. This may sound like a lot, but they only take seconds to do.

- Begin by simply squeezing and releasing the PC muscle. The PC muscle is part of the group of muscles that are used to stop the flow of urine. You can locate this muscle by first practicing with actually stopping the flow of urine. It is good to isolate this muscle from the rectal muscle that is used in the deer exercise.
- In time, you will be able to slow down the squeezing of this muscle and hold the squeeze for a few seconds. Sets can be done off and on throughout your day. As you slow down and intensify the squeeze, you can perform fewer repetitions.

The younger that we start these practices, the better. Ideally, do not wait until after childbirth or when issues arise. These are easy muscles to keep strong and healthy. Dedicate a little time as often as possible to practice. Feeling jubilant and sexy nourishes the essence of our youthfulness and self-expression.

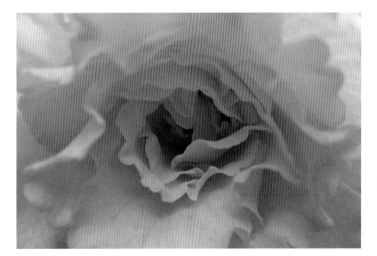

Love is the answer,
but while you are waiting for the answer,
sex raises some pretty good questions.
~ Woody Allen

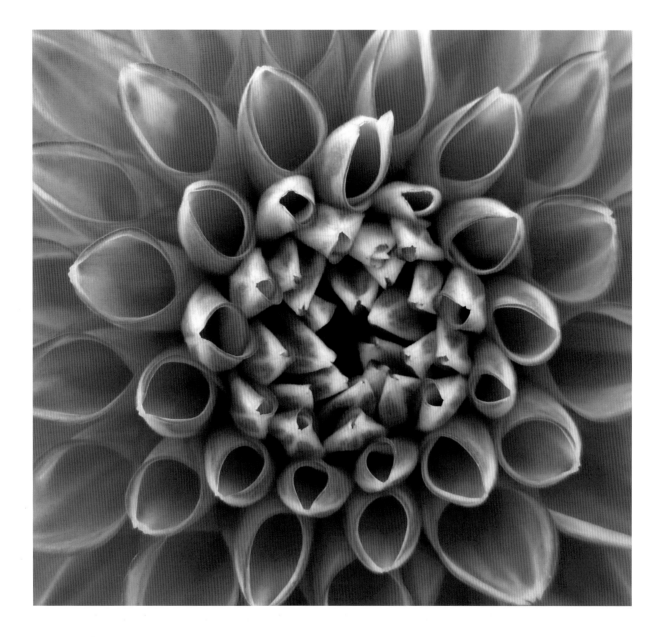

We will discover the nature of our particular genius
when we stop trying to conform to our own or to other people's models,
learn to be ourselves, and allow our natural channel to open.

– SHAKTI GAWAIN

for sweetness…

Meditation in Motion:
mind & body in rhythm

The Benefits of a Quiet Mind

– Deepak Chopra, international lecturer and author of more than 50 books on mind-body healing, estimates that people who regularly meditate often have a biological age that is between 5 and 10 years lower than their actual age.

– While you sleep, your oxygen usage drops 8%. During a meditation session, it can drop 10 to 20%. Muscles that are used in dream states relax during meditation.

– Hormones with a calming effect like melatonin and serotonin increase as a result of meditating. The stress hormone cortisol decreases.

– Meditating has a positive effect on our sense of hearing, our blood pressure and our eyesight.

– People who meditate recover more quickly from diseases and usually experience situations as less stressful.

These are only a few of the many benefits of meditation. Research scientists agree unanimously that stress plays a significant role in our emotional and physical aging process, and meditation is known to release stress.

Dan Buettner, author of *The Blue Zone,* traveled the globe to research the similarities of centenarians, people who live over 100 years. Meditation and prayer were two of the healthful living components the centenarians shared. Mr. Buettner believes that by making lifestyle changes, an additional ten years can be added to many people's lives.

Meditation has been described as anything that can completely bring us into the present moment, and keep us present. There are numerous techniques to achieve mindfulness, most of which have existed for thousands of years. It is wise to explore options for achieving mindfulness to determine what is the best for you. Jon Kabat-Zinn, a leader in mindfulness practices, has written a number of best-selling books on the subject.

Moving Meditation

Most people imagine having to sit cross-legged on the floor, unmoving, as a means to achieve inner stillness. The good news for people who may view sitting still as an insurmountable challenge is that you do not have to sit still in order to achieve mindfulness and greater well-being.

Inviting spontaneous movement, or moving meditation, is by far, a lesser-known form of meditation, yet anyone can do this. There are no rules, simply quiet your mind, and open your body to natural movement.

The added benefit of bringing spontaneous movement into your meditation time is that your body is simultaneously able to access healing and rejuvenation. This healing is not something that you can access from your mind or from sources outside of your body. As you move into a deeper, meditative state you can awaken your inner wisdom, often referred to spirit, subconscious or your infinite well within.

At first, it may feel contrived and anything but natural. The more we quiet our mind so that we are not judging our movements, the richer and more satisfying our practice becomes. Dr. Tienko Ting, the founder of Natural Chi Movement, and author of *Natural Chi Movement: Accessing the World of the Miraculous* shares his thoughts:

"I have seen many people who practice Natural Chi Movement heal themselves of all manner of physical illness and open themselves without effort to spiritual enlightenment. If you are trying to get something from a physical source, there will always be limitations. Physical energy is found only within physical bodies. It is limited. In contrast, spiritual energy is everywhere, and it is limitless. Tapping into spiritual energy is the only way we can get at an unlimited source of energy."

I'm going out to find myself, but if I return before I get back, please hold me until I get there.

- FROM CALVIN AND HOBBES

Depending on our age, our bodies range from being made up of 60% to 79% water. We are naturally fluid, though in childhood we have often been told to sit still. As adults, there are even greater cultural restraints on moving our bodies. Consequently, we suppress much of our natural desire to move. When we invite spontaneous movement to occur in our body, it is as if we are re-learning what is innate. It is a divine right to honor, access and use this energy and wisdom.

It is not necessary to have any warm-up, or preparation. Initially, some people feel a simple chi exercise is helpful. Over time, you may find that your desire to intuitively move naturally arises throughout your day. There are no right or wrong ways and you can practice as long as you desire. People in the East practice spontaneous chi for an hour or more a day. I find that fifteen minutes every morning is a great way to start my day.

Spontaneous movement enables us to connect with our inner wisdom and true nature. It is this energy that becomes our guide, rather than our mind, or someone else's.

Getting Started

"You know how we lose ourselves in an interesting story until our surroundings are completely obliterated — that is concentration — and we can so train ourselves to meditate that we immerse our minds in our subject to the exclusion of everything else."

– DR. VENICE BLOODWORTH, KEY TO YOURSELF

Most people find this practice brings a sense of freedom. Be patient with yourself. Just as with sitting meditation, thoughts will come to mind in the beginning. Your mind may question whether your movements are premeditated or spontaneous. In time, the chatter and questioning subside and you find yourself effortlessly, fluidly moving. Keep coming back into your breath. If it is helpful, repeat the words, *"I am breathing in, I am breathing out."*

Empty your bladder before you begin. You can practice standing, sitting or lying down. I find standing to be the best way to begin. As you practice, you may be drawn to change positions. Occasionally you may feel a need to lie down. Consciously move wherever you feel drawn and then sink back into your breath and allow your movements to begin again. This practice requires you to open to receive and to trust in yourself.

Occasionally, emotions arise. We are of body, mind and spirit. Our emotions range from pure joy and freedom, to deep sadness and tears. Go with the flow, knowing that at any time, you can stop and begin your practice again at a later time.

Practicing first thing in the morning is a great time to move with all of nature rising. As with sitting meditation, it is often easier to maintain a quiet mind before engaging in the fullness of our daily lives. As with all of the Fountain of Youth exercises, practicing outside whenever possible is ideal. Being barefoot on the earth is even better. In China, it is common to see many people in the parks practicing a variety of chi exercises every morning.

Warming Up... into Infinity

If you would like an exercise to engage yourself in moving meditation, this Infinity Chi Kung exercise is very soothing and centering.

- From standing, focus on your breath. Close your eyes and bring your attention inward.
- Some people imagine a single flame, and bring their undivided attention to that flame. Another option is to bring your attention to your forehead, or third eye point. You may also wish to bring to mind the image of a multi-petaled flower, like a lotus or rose.
- Fix your attention on something singular. Pause here for a few breaths. This practice in yoga is often referred to as centering, and usually enables one to begin becoming more present.
- Next, bring your awareness to the soles of your feet. Notice if your weight is centered; if not, center your weight by adjusting how you stand.

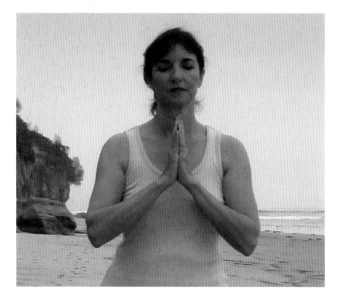

Model: *Marla Daigh, 56 years young.*

- Then, imagine drawing a figure eight, or infinity symbol, with your hips or the soles of your feet.
- Roll your weight back on the outside of your right foot, up through the inside of your right foot, roll back on the outside of your left foot, around the heel, and up through the inside of your left foot. Your whole body will gently flow with this movement. Repeat as long as you like.

You can also explore the opposite direction. Roll your weight forward on the outside of your right foot, down through the inside of your right foot, around your left heel, up through the outside of your left foot and down the inside of your left foot. Continue repeating.

One direction may feel more natural than the other. In the East, rolling backward on the outside the foot is considered more yin (feminine or contemplative), and rolling forward on the outside of the foot is more yang (masculine or expressive). This exercise can bring balance to a tendency of being either more yang or more yin.

- Feel free to drop your gaze toward the floor, or close your eyes. Allow your arms to hang loosely at your sides.
- As you breathe, you may have a gentle awareness of how fluid your body is. Continue as long as desired.

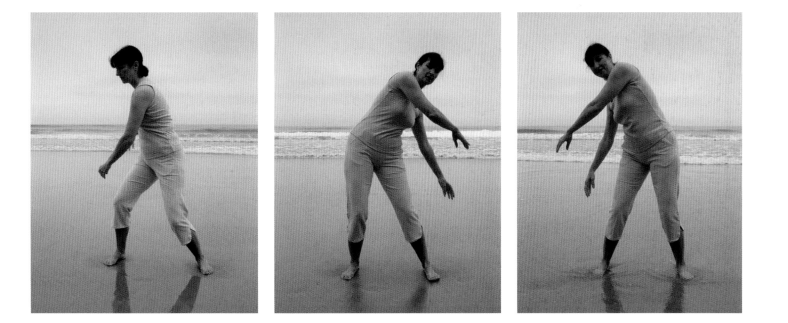

Your Chi Movement

Eventually, allow yourself to lose a distinction of when conscious warming-up ends, and your inner energy or natural chi takes over. It is often like a dance, as you flow between your mind leading, and then you surrender again, and are led in ways that you could not imagine. Keep bringing your attention back to your breath as needed, and trust.

When I began Natural Chi Movement with Dr. Ting, the first thing I became aware of was my baby finger moving! It was subtle. Fortunately, I had quieted my mind long enough to realize that this movement had started. I was fascinated, for I knew my mind could never have thought of this motion. Other subtle movements began to flow into larger movements. I was a believer from that moment.

Your practice will evolve and change, though usually, there are repetitious patterns that can occur until your inner energy has healed or rejuvenated the places it was drawn to move toward.

Meditation, both in stillness and in motion, are practices I do every day. As Jon Kabat-Zinn so eloquently stated, "In the stillness of formal practice, we do turn our energies inward, only to discover that we contain the entire world in our own mind and body." Within that world is, unquestionably, a key to longevity.

TIP: You may find it helpful to set a timer so that you are free to truly sink into your practice.

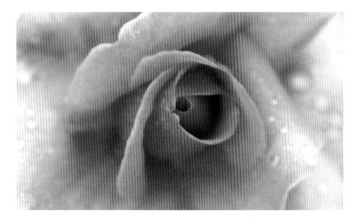

When you take a flower in your hand and really look at it,
it's your world for the moment.
~ GEORGIA O'KEEFFE

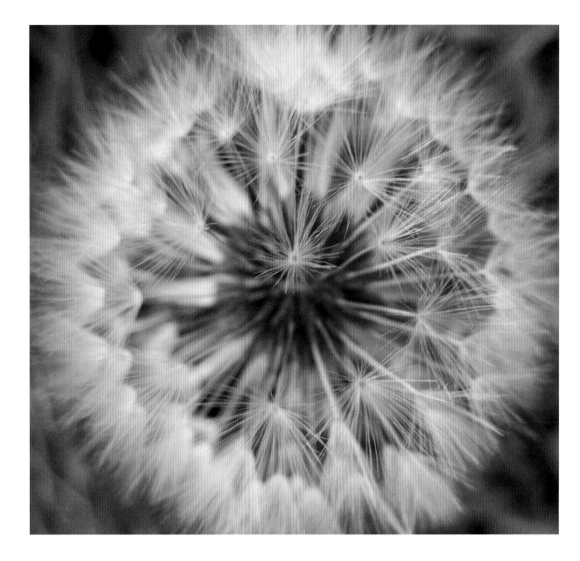

Inside your body there are flowers.
One flower has a thousand petals.
That will do for a place to sit.
Sitting there you will have a glimpse
of beauty inside the body and out of it,
before gardens and after gardens.

~ KABIR

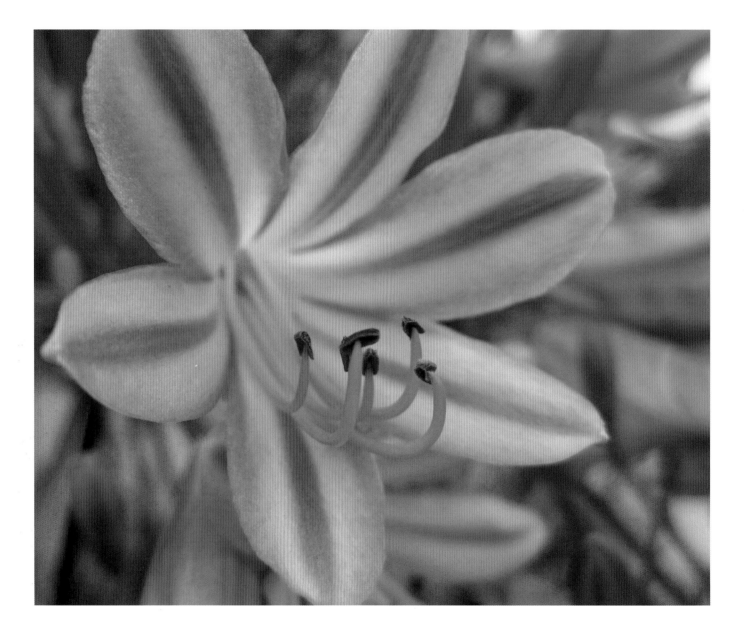

Be faithful in small things
because it is in them
that your strength lies.

~ MOTHER TERESA

your daily bread...

Longevity of Body: caring for your temple

Essentials on the Inside

Throughout time, people have revered the human body as a temple, a home for their spirit, choosing and orchestrating daily activities steeped from this belief. When we prioritize the care and feeding of our body, mind and spirit, every aspect of our life can flow with more energy, radiance and ease.

Exercise is only one ingredient in the longevity recipe. Our every thought and action creates an equal or greater reaction that will affect our future. How you think and feel about creating your well-being will determine the success of your outcome. I embrace caring for my body like an artist creating her masterpiece. The clay is in my hands to sculpt. The gifts of the earth are opportunities that we are each given. Everything I take into my body, from the air above to the water below, affects the outcome of my recipe.

Embracing a Fountain of Youth lifestyle can be an adventure, one that may stretch your muscles and beliefs in ways you didn't know existed, broadening every horizon. In hindsight, many of us have broadened our beliefs and understandings about food and lifestyle as we have evolved. It is time for us to listen to our bodies, to acknowledge what is most important for us, to redefine what nourishes our *whole* being, to awaken our minds and enliven our spirits.

FRESH AIR

Our bodies thrive on fresh air. As architectural advancements create more energy-efficient homes and buildings, recycled air is a usual by-product. A key to the well-being of your temple is to keep doors and windows open as much as possible. Spend time outside in nature daily, infusing your body with fresh air. Being near forests, especially old-growth trees, or surrounded by the beauty and radiance of flowers, will enliven your every breath.

Most building materials, finishes, carpeting and furnishings are toxic and will outgas for years. Quite often people feel ill, or are prone to excessive illnesses, in new homes and offices, and they never make the connection. Our immune system can be compromised by constantly having to work harder due to indoor contaminants. These products also end up as environmental waste hazards.

Take time to educate yourself about healthy products for greener living spaces. This includes the time that you are sleeping. We spend many hours a day in bed and unless you have purchased an organic, natural bed, you are breathing in chemical toxins while you sleep.

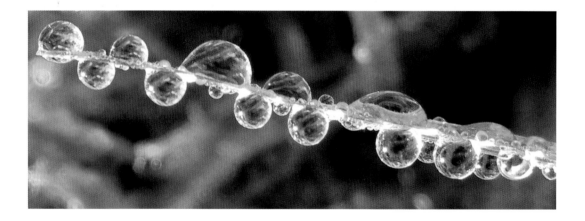

HYDRATING WITH WATER

Pure water is the most important refreshment in life. As a general rule, if a person eats a Standard American Diet (SAD), they need to drink approximately half of their body weight in ounces per day. For example, if you weigh 120 pounds, you would consume approximately 60 ounces of water. If your diet is rich in raw fruits and vegetables or juices, this amount can be reduced.

Water is the only drink for a wise man.

- HENRY DAVID THOREAU

Dehydration is a leading cause in a number of diseases and premature aging — and it can raise stress hormone levels. Often people overeat, thinking they are hungry, when in actuality they are thirsty. It is usually helpful to measure your water intake to be certain you're getting your recommended daily intake. Other liquids do *not* hydrate the body the way water does, and caffeinated beverages act as diuretics.

TIP: A squeeze of fresh organic lemon juice in your water can help curb your appetite and alkalize your body.

Choose your water consciously. If you drink tap water, or purified water, educate yourself about the water. It is scientifically proven that numerous contaminants and pharmaceuticals *cannot* be removed from recycled tap and toilet water. If you wish to truly radiate vitality and you live in an urban area, it is wise to purchase the best *spring or artesian* water, or a quality filtration system. Bathing and showering in fluoridated water is also a hazard. Please take time to educate yourself about the misconceptions surrounding the benefits of fluoride as well as the health risks of plastics.

FOOD FOR LONGEVITY

It can be daunting to attempt figuring out how to educate oneself about nutrition. What is "best" can change with every internet site or talk show host, though for the first time in years there is growing agreement about the basics of good nutrition. Even the FDA has announced that a plant-based diet is the healthiest option. Freeing the body of saturated fats, preservatives, growth hormones, red meat, chemicals, cooked oils, excessive carbohydrates, processed foods, corn syrup and sugar is recognized as necessary for health and longevity. In essence, get back to basics. You are what you eat.

"Let thy food by thy medicine and thy medicine be thy food."

- HIPPOCRATES

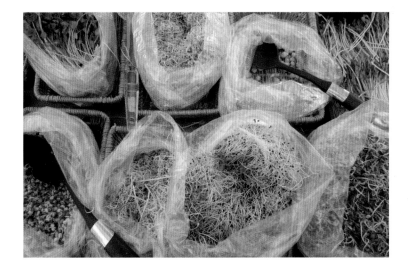

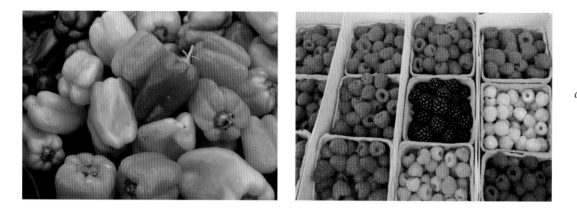

An anti-inflammatory diet that includes a minimum of 50% to 70 % raw food can provide vital enzymes for digestion while greatly improving our health and enhancing our youthful radiance. The quality of our air, soil and water is constantly changing. Choosing organic foods, free from pesticides, growth hormones, GMOs and chemicals is always the best choice for your longevity.

Making healthier nutritional choices can immediately reduce or eliminate health concerns and symptoms. These include numerous diseases, obesity, skin outbreaks, inflammation, chronic pain, headache, allergies and high blood pressure.

Diseases, such as cancer, need an acid host. The addition of leafy green, nutrient-rich foods, which help create an alkaline environment, works wonders in maintaining our ph balance. Regularly seasoning with a few readily available herbs, such as turmeric, garlic, ginger and cinnamon, among others, helps to reduce inflammation and support the immune system.

Diseases, such as diabetes, the disease that The American Diabetes Association claims to be "incurable," are in fact, *curable* through a live, plant-based diet and holistic approach. Please refer to Dr. Gabriel Cousins, *There is a Cure for Diabetes,* book in Resources. More information is also included on diet-based cancer therapies.

Occasionally, the effects of the foods that we eat are not subtle. The more consciously you choose your nutrition, the more sensitive your body will become. Upon changing from the SAD to more healthful eating, you can begin to feel the effects of foods to which you were desensitized, if you choose to consume them.

The effects of your dietary choices on your body are even more heightened after a cleanse or fast. Not only do our organs work less strenuously and more efficiently, there is also an anti-aging hormone in our body that is produced more efficiently when we fast. There is abundant evidence to prove that fasting contributes to a longer life.

TIP: Studies have also shown that eating fresh, live foods from every color of the rainbow can contribute to our longevity.

Educate yourself about healthier foods and then focus on developing your will "muscle." We tend not to view our will as a muscle, but it is one we can strengthen with daily practice. Choose foods that you can feel good about eating. Feeling regret after eating an extra dessert, or a less-than-excellent choice, can further challenge your body to properly digest. Trust your choices as you strive to develop your will and your knowledge about food.

A good time to begin exercising that will muscle is at the market. Choose the foods that land in your cart wisely. Also, choosing to shop in health food stores and at local farmer's markets instead of grocery stores can facilitate your transitioning to a healthier, more alkalizing, cuisine — you often feel better just by being there!

Whatever you take in, be grateful for it. Once something crosses the threshold of your lips, it is a part of who you are. It is creating the quality of your life; for better or worse, you are wedded to the energy and the effect.

OUR RADIO DIALS

Food takes on many forms. The books we read, the television programs and films we watch, the sounds and aromas… every choice you make throughout your day will contribute, in one way or the other, to the quality and length of your life.

Imagine that everything is energy, and all energy has a vibration. Food is similar to a radio; every food has a different frequency or station. Some are "higher" frequencies on the dial than others. You may notice that if you experiment with making healthier choices toward a plant-based diet that other foods lose their appeal. It is as though you tune your radio dial to a different station.

To lengthen thy life, lessen thy meals. The best of all medicines are rest and fasting.

- BENJAMIN FRANKLIN

Just as the crashing waves caress the beach cliffs every day, every night, relentlessly, and thus shapes those cliffs ever so subtly, so too do the foods we eat shape our forms subtly, slowly and methodically over time.

- DAVID WOLFE, CREATOR OF LONGEVITY NOW AND ONE OF AMERICA'S FOREMOST NUTRITION EXPERTS.

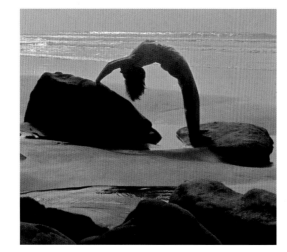

Essentials on the Outside

CLEANSING WITH WATER

Water is just as healing and cleansing outside your body as it is to drink. Any time you feel upset, stressed or unable to clearly think through a situation, step into the shower or bath. Feel the cleansing power of water. If a shower isn't possible, lie down for a minute and visualize a waterfall washing over and through you, washing away your tension, stress or negative feelings. Some spiritual practices advocate taking showers upon rising and before retiring to sleep. This can help you to be more present to your day, and to sleep better at night after washing away the day.

Warm baths infused with essential oils, such as lavender, have a deeply calming effect. Being able to jump into the ocean or be in fresh water in nature is ideal for washing away the stress of modern life. Stress is one of the greatest contributors to premature aging. Make the effort to find ways to de-stress, to clear away unwanted thoughts and emotions as soon as they arise, to keep yourself more present and youthful.

The greatest wealth is health.
– VIRGIL

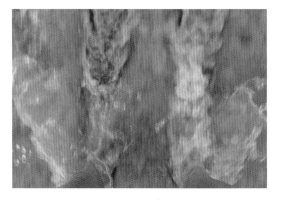

NOURISHING OUR LARGEST ORGAN

Skin is our largest organ and everything that we put onto our skin contributes to its vitality and radiance. When you look in the mirror and see healthy glowing skin, you feel more youthful! Again, getting back to basics is the healthiest choice. Everything that you put onto your skin is in essence feeding your skin.

If you wish to nourish your skin from the inside out, lecithin, essential fatty acids, Omega oils, dark leafy greens, berries and raw cacao (chocolate) will all improve the look, feel and vitality of your skin. Juice from the aloe vera plant is also available for internal consumption.

It is found in health food stores and is known to contain amino acids, vital minerals like calcium and magnesium, enzymes, vitamins, polysaccharides, nitrogen and other components. It is also known for aiding arthritis, decreasing cholesterol levels, stabilizing blood sugar, and healing the lining of the stomach and intestines.

Fresh aloe leaves can be found in health food stores and provide one of the best foods for the body. For the skin, aloe vera gel is widely recognized as an aid for sunburn, though cosmetic and health-related industries are discovering numerous additional benefits. Ideally, use fresh, raw gel on your skin daily. If you purchase a commercially packaged gel, please read the ingredients.

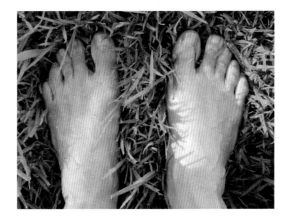

NATURALLY EXFOLIATE & INVIGORATE

TIP: Walk outside in the dew-covered grass in your bare feet. Find a safe spot, free from obstacles and pet use. Breathe deeply as you slowly invigorate your soles and rejuvenate your spirit! Even a few focused minutes can enliven your day. If there are affirmations or visualizations you like, bring those to mind while you walk. Choose how your day will blossom!

For centuries, dry brushing the skin has been used to exfoliate, prevent dry skin and stimulate beautiful skin renewal. The skin is known as the third kidney, daily eliminating and detoxing one quarter of the body's waste. It is the last organ to receive nutrients.

Through dry brushing we can accelerate detoxification, increase circulation and remove dead skin layers and cellulite. This practice helps to prevent premature aging, strengthen the immune system, cleanse the lymphatic system and stimulate our hormone glands. Overall, you are left with an invigorated and refreshed feeling. Loofahs or dry brushes are available in health food stores and drug stores.

Sea salt scrubs offer many of the same benefits of dry brushing. It is a little more complex to do, especially over your entire body. I often focus on my feet and find that alone to be very revitalizing. Getting circulation to our feet is crucial. The feet are the farthest from your heart, so it is natural that your blood flow is not as strong on its own here. Your whole body benefits from attention that you give to your feet.

When you shower, at the end switch the faucet to cold. This will help further increase circulation in the skin and it's very invigorating! Once you are out of the shower, remember that the products you put on your skin are food for your skin. Choose organic, chemical-free products. Edgar Cayce, along with other leaders in the health field, advocates only putting pure oils on our skin—oils that you would consume internally, such as coconut or cocoa butters.

*Our bodies
are our gardens —
our wills
are our gardeners.*

– *WILLIAM
SHAKESPEARE*

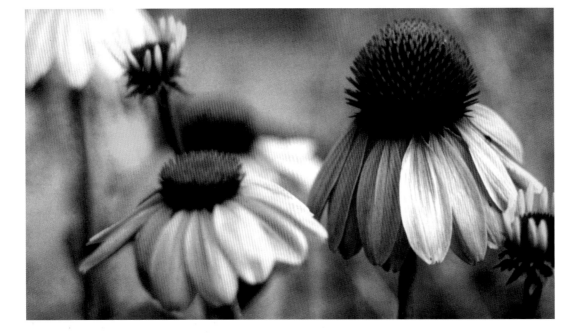

EARLY TO BED, EARLY TO RISE

Age-old wisdom still holds true. We know that digestion takes time. The earlier we can eat dinner, the better. This enables the body to thoroughly complete digestion and relax into restoration. The largest meal, or significant protein intake of your day, is best consumed by midday. Strive to wind down your evening as early as possible; the less stimulation the better. Replicate the natural world by lessening sounds, dimming your lights and engaging in relaxing activities.

Chinese medicine practitioners advocate being asleep before 10 o'clock to fully nourish the body's internal clock. From 10 pm to 2 am is when the body's immune system replenishes. It is also believed that removing all jewelry from the body facilitates the unimpeded flow of chi throughout the night.

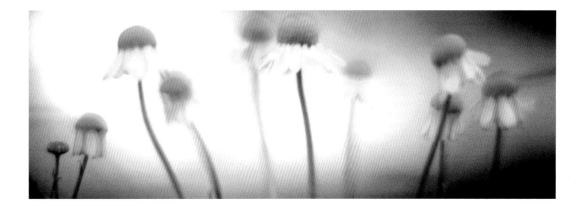

Normally, the best position for your spine is to sleep on your back. Use only a soft pillow to support your neck, not your head. You may also experiment with a rolled blanket or small pillow under your knees. If you currently sleep on your belly, lie down on your back with a wall of pillows around both sides of your body before going to sleep. It can take a few nights, but eventually you can break the habit of turning over to sleep on your belly. This position creates added weight and stress on all of your organs. If you sleep on your left side, you are adding extra stress to your heart all night. If you need to sleep on your side, make it your right.

If snoring complicates a sound night's sleep for you or your spouse, explore changes to your diet, including the elimination of dairy, flour and processed foods. Eating ice cream or other cold sweets can interrupt your sleep and often negatively influence your dreams, making it even more difficult to achieve sound sleep. Keeping a window open near your bed will enable you to benefit from breathing in more chi. Even in the freezing cold winters of upstate New York, I kept my bedroom window open a small crack. Especially in colder climates, the air in homes can become very dry.

STEP BY STEP

As with all exercises, outdoors is best. Throughout my day, I often take breaks from being at my desk to go outside and walk around the neighborhood. If you walk 30 minutes a day, studies show measurable increase in your life expectancy.

When we walk outdoors there is always something new to listen to, to see or to smell. I always feel refreshed and renewed even after a fifteen-minute jaunt around my neighborhood. I often take my camera and photograph flowers and nature. Most of the nature photographs in this book were taken on my morning walks. Your daily walk can double as an important dose of your "sunshine" vitamin.

It is reported in the Archives of Internal Medicine that those with the lowest Vitamin D levels have more than double the risk of dying from heart disease and other causes. Vitamin D is crucial to our well-being. Expose as much of your body to the sun as possible, avoiding the hours of 11 to 3. New studies are finding that additional supplementation of Vitamin D may be necessary.

OTHER ESSENTIALS

There are a few other foundational practices for longevity of body that I feel are instrumental and worthy of note. One is the use of essential oils, which can add years to your life. Whether it's in your bathtub, as a natural perfume on your body, or in an aromatherapy diffuser in your house or car, oils can relax, purify and energize you and your environment. Health food stores offer tester bottles so you can choose the ones that resonate with you.

Another helpful tool is using rebounders, the small trampolines that are made for indoors. Alternative cancer clinics, especially for women with breast cancer, make rebounding part of daily therapy to oxygenate the lymph system. Studies have shown that moderate rebounding for a few minutes a day can significantly increase the effectiveness of the lymph system along with numerous other health benefits. For information on rebounders visit www.needak.com.

Lastly, remember that color is therapy, and invite color into your life. In the same way that our body can benefit from consuming an array of colors, our spirit can also soar with the addition of radiant colors in our clothes and in our homes. Express your true self, and delight in adorning your body and living space with organic fibers, aromas and gems of the earth that give you joy and pleasure.

Our outer body reflects our inner body. Cleanse and honor your temple inside and out. Take time to educate yourself and make the changes that are right for you. Please visit *www. naomicall.com* for further information.

I often observe in fasting participants that… concentration seems to improve,
creative thinking expands, depression lifts, insomnia stops, anxieties fade,
the mind becomes more tranquil, and a natural joy begins to appear…
when the physical toxins are cleared from the brain cells, mind-brain function
automatically and significantly improves, and spiritual capacities expand.

~ GABRIEL COUSENS, M.D. FOUNDER OF TREE OF LIFE REJUVENATION CENTER

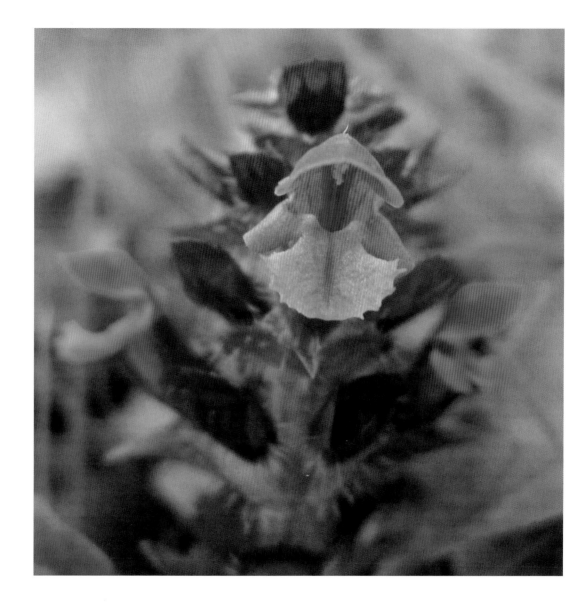

*A wise man should consider that health is the greatest of human blessings,
and learn how by his own thought to derive benefit from his illnesses.*

~ HIPPOCRATES

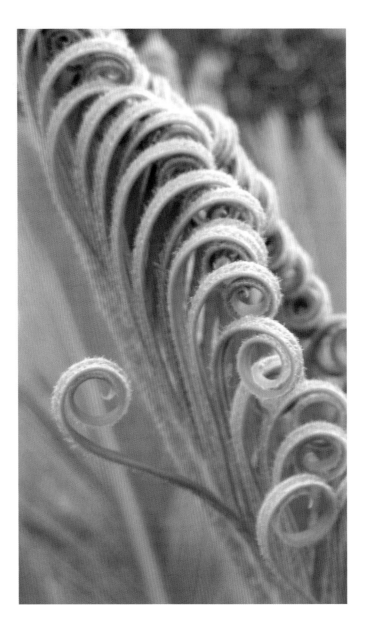

"We are the product of our prevailing habits of thought.
Each is building his own world from within;
thought is the builder…
every experience with which you meet has been built
for you by your own interior thought processes."

— **DR. VENICE BLOODWORTH,** *FROM KEY TO YOURSELF*

sharpen your utensil…

Longevity of Mind: using your wisdom

There is universal agreement that a key to vital longevity is active engagement of our brain. Our brains need exercise. It is recommended that every day we change up our routines, break our habits and make concerted efforts to create new challenges for ourselves. Following are some commonly recognized exercises for increasing brain power:

– Take up bridge, study a foreign language or anything that you want to learn.
– Read and play music. Classical music will challenge your brain the most.
– Do games, word puzzles and math problems.
– Read often, on a wide variety of stimulating topics.
– Engage in conversations that will take you out of your comfort zone.
– Take on memorizing everyday things, like a grocery list, poem or saying.
– Study a new word every day.
– Alternate using your non-dominant hand.

"As long as you can see each day as a chance
for something new to happen,
something you never experienced before,
you will stay young."

~ SADIE DELANY

Nourishing the Brain

The brain, just like the rest of your body, benefits from deep breathing, meditation and a healthy diet. Foods rich in omega fatty acids such as hemp, flax and pumpkin seeds nourish brain function. Omegas are also found in fish, though it's important to research the source of the fish and make choices that are low in mercury. Smaller fish, which are lower on the food chain, are usually healthier choices. Increase your memory, not your toxicity.

Educate yourself about the sources of all of your food, especially meats and dairy. These foods, if not labeled organic, often contain growth hormones, and are raised in horrid conditions that create devastating environmental imbalances. It is best to choose wild caught, rather than farm-raised fish, and free-range meat, poultry and dairy The energy of the food you consume affects the quality of your thoughts. The quality of your thoughts affects the quality of your life.

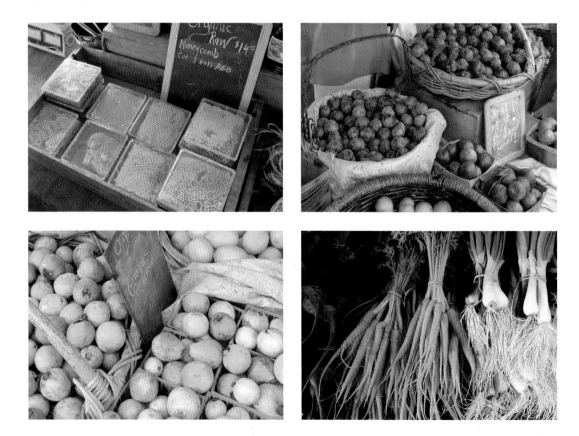

What We Think, We Become

AFFIRMATIONS & VISUALIZATION

Every thought we think is creating our future.

~ LOUISE L. HAY

Your mind is your most powerful tool. When we harness the power of our thoughts and direct the mind onto a path free from fear, life can flow with greater ease. Affirmations and positive thoughts can be a very useful tool for manifesting the life you desire.

Often, affirmations begin with the words, *"I am...."*. From there, fill in the blanks, then fill your house and car with post-its to remind yourself. The bathroom mirror is a great place to post an affirmation. The next step is to fill your heart with the feelings that you would feel if the object of your desire were already so. For example, if you create the affirmation, *"I am youthful, radiant and beautiful,"* feel youthful, radiant and beautiful as you say those words. See yourself in the mirror exactly as you wish. Then affirm... and so it is.

Throughout your day affirm, over and over, that which you desire. When we work with the subconscious it can take time, so please be patient. Your mind is a powerful tool, it is crucial for you to gain control of your thoughts and to recognize the law of attraction. For some, visualizing imagery is more powerful than words. Give each approach time to get to know what is best for you.

Courage and faith in yourself is greatly enhanced through daily affirmations and visualizations. Create in your inner world, building a strong foundation from within.

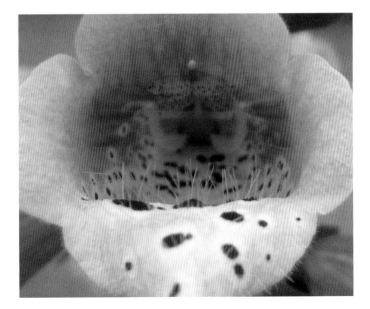

DECISION-MAKING MADE SIMPLE

It is also important to not hold regrets or worry about our choices. Once you make a decision, let it go. Trust that it was best and stay in the present. Don't second-guess yourself, or spend precious energy wishing you had made a different choice in your life previous to this moment. Worry and fear stress the body; and reliving the past makes it impossible to truly be present and can greatly impede and undermine your efforts toward longevity.

"If it is not a yes, it's a no."

Embracing these simple words has proven to be a real time and energy saver in my life. I used to deliberate in grey spaces, and now, if something truly resonates within me; it's a yes. If it doesn't, I let it go and trust that it will come back if it is meant to be.

When decisions do not feel simple and clear, muscle testing, a simplified form of body movement, can be a useful tool. Muscle testing, also known as kinesiology, is a simple way that you can check your muscle strength as a tool to access your deepest reaction to a concept or object. Information on my website (*www.naomicall.com*) can help you learn how to deepen your relationship with your body's wisdom. Many health practitioners use kinesiology to fine tune and maximize their clients' results. It enables you to access the infinite storehouse of wisdom within you to help guide your decision-making.

Your imagination is your preview of life's coming attractions.

- ALBERT EINSTEIN

Words to Live By

Simply stated, what we put our attention on thrives, for better or worse. Buddha said: "Think as though your every thought were to be etched in fire across the sky for all and everything to see."

I believe this quote has impacted my life more than any other. I grew up thinking that my thoughts were my private world, that what we thought had no impact on anyone or anything. I have profound gratitude to Buddha for bringing a new paradigm to light.

Life is significantly different when we truly embrace that our thoughts, not just our actions, impact the world around us. People often do not think of their thoughts as things that can create beauty and peace, or chaos and conflict. Now I understand: of course they can.

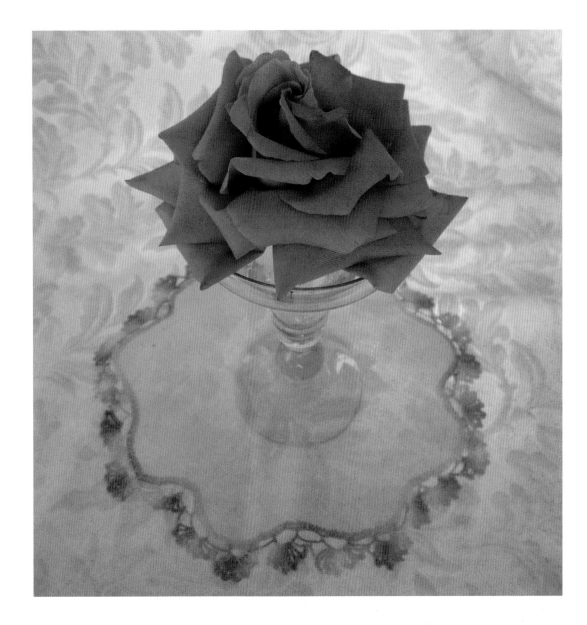

You can choose to see your glass as half empty, or half full…
or, you could choose to see your glass as overflowing.
To some, overflowing might appear as a mess…
to others, a thing of beauty.

~ NAOMI CALL

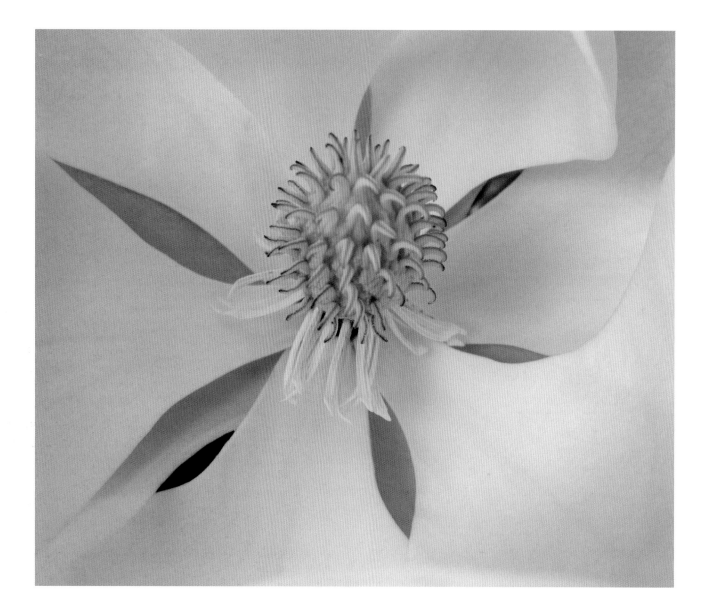

Stop the words now.
Open the window in the center of your chest,
and let spirit move in and out.
Let yourself be silently drawn
by the stronger pull of what you really love.

- RUMI

a sprinkle of love…

Longevity of Spirit: connecting with your heart

Being in our true essence and joy is what feeds our heart — this is the key ingredient in our longevity recipe. Do what you love, go where you love, and be with the people, animals and nature that you love to be with…. and you will … be radiantly youthful.

Follow your bliss, for being happy is what keeps us healthy. The truth is, people who are happy rarely get sick. It is not too late to explore, without further hesitation, that which you have not yet done.

Singing, dancing, painting or any artistic activity that you enjoy can satiate your soul and spirit the way that water satiates your cells, creating a deeper sense of wholeness and well-being. People often exclaim that they are not artists. You don't have to be an "artist;" *everyone is an artist of something, including themselves and their life.*

Our spirits yearn for creative expression. It may take a few trials to become clear what your form of self-expression is. Engaging your creativity will add years of joy and newfound energy to your life!

Exercises for the Spirit

There are a few longevity exercises that I feel are helpful for connecting us to our heart, to each other, and to universal energy.

ENERGIZING THE HEART

Taoists practice an exercise they refer to as Energizing the Heart. It is performed from standing or sitting.

- Bring your palms together and vigorously rub for a few seconds, warming the hands.
- Draw your arms up, elbows bent with your fingertips almost touching in front of your heart.
- Bring a soft focus to the tips of your fingers, or better yet, close your eyes.
- Breathe deeply and open yourself to feeling the energy that is radiating from the tips of your fingers, into your heart, strengthening your heart and the surrounding vessels before flowing out again.

Be Patient. With persistence and a quiet mind you can begin to feel the tingling of energy from your fingertips. As you do, affirm the increased flow of chi to your heart, even if you do not yet feel it.

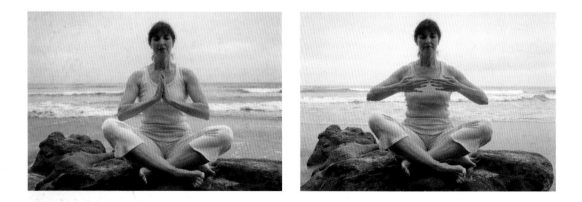

If it is helpful to bring in a visual to quiet your mind, experiment with focusing on a blossoming flower. Feel your heart blossoming into fullness, becoming stronger, as your energy flows through.

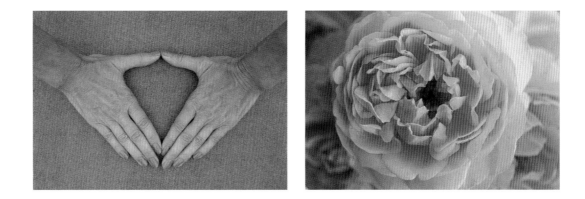

As we work with Do-In and chi practices, our chi builds and becomes stronger in our bodies.

SUN SALUTE (AKA IN HONOR)

Ideally, this exercise is performed outside directly on the earth, though it can be modified to be done anywhere. This is an ancient ritual that was often done first thing, before all other exercises. I have found it to be wonderful ritual to bookend my day, or my practice. This is completely different than the popular sun salutation that is done in yoga.

- In Honor is done by bringing your body into a *seiza*, or child pose.
- Bring the tips of your thumbs together and the sides of your index fingers, creating a triangle. Rest your palms down on the earth in this position at forehead height.
- Bow forward, so that your forehead, or third eye point, may rest within the triangle.
- Drop into your breath. Pause here as long as you wish. When you are ready to release, press your palms down as you inhale up.

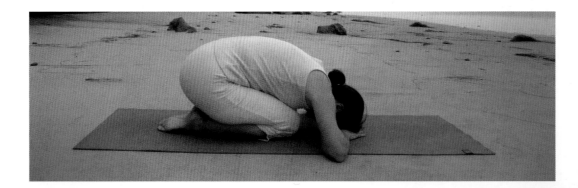

MODIFICATIONS: This can also be performed on your bed in the morning. Feel free to use stacked pillows to rest your hands upon so that your forehead may meet your hands and be cradled. You can also rest pillows on your heels to support your tailbone.

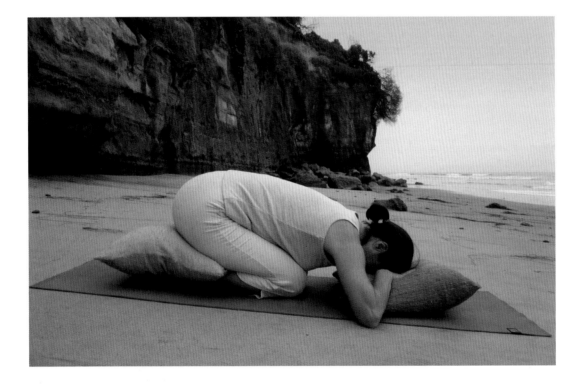

Early practitioners believed that, in resting their forehead upon the earth, they were connecting their third eye chakra, or energy center, to the earth. In doing so, they knew that they were creating a connection with every other living thing on the planet. I also feel that this exercise can help you to clear your mind, allowing thoughts and worries to be absorbed by the earth. Most people experience a deepened peace and sense of connection. For some, it becomes a beautiful gateway into meditation or a wonderful way to start the day.

The gesture of bowing oneself forward in reverence is in itself a profound act.

Model: *Marla Daigh, 56 years young.*

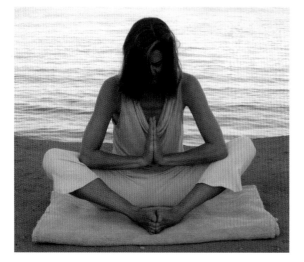

TIP: It is lovely to draw your palms and soles together. Feel the warmth of connecting. Soften your gaze or close your eyes, and feel your inner radiance. If your soles do not meet, visualize the connection.

The Journey

Sipping from the Fountain of Youth is a journey. One that begins with connecting with ourselves. For it is here that we can dip into an infinite well of wisdom. There is indeed a Fountain of Youth deep within your body, your mind and your spirit. It is up to you to believe, to choose to look inside of yourself, versus outside. The Fountain of Youth elixir is your life essence, your passion and joy, your choice and creation.

Be in the driver's seat of your life. Every day is a gift. How we see, think and feel about the world, and how youthful and joyful we feel, are moment by moment choices.

Each breath is a new moment that will never happen again. See the beauty in it, smell it, taste it, touch it, breathe it.... be alive with the gift and love of life.

Be in your beauty with a childlike wonder of life, see everything as new again... with gratitude and joy. The possibilities are endless... as is your life.

The only way to live is to accept each minute as an unrepeatable miracle,
which is exactly what it is: a miracle and unrepeatable.

~ STORM JAMESON

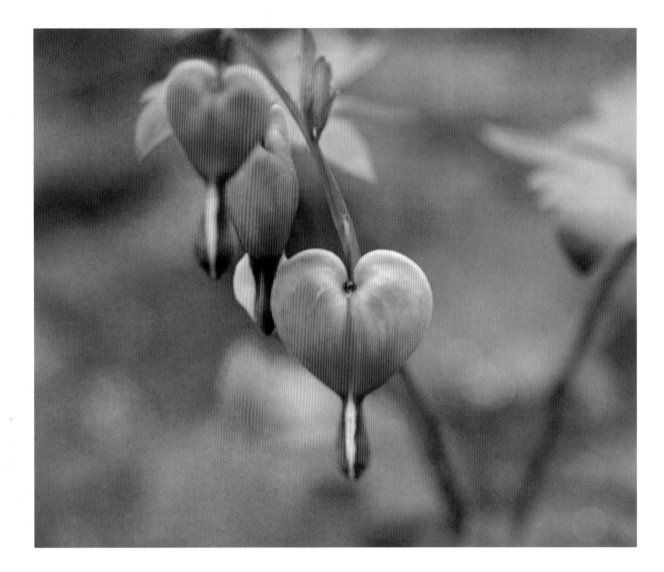

Gratitude unlocks the fullness of life.
It turns what we have into enough, and more.
It turns denial into acceptance, chaos to order, confusion to clarity.
It can turn a meal into a feast, a house into a home,
a stranger into a friend.
Gratitude makes sense of our past, brings peace for today,
and creates a vision for tomorrow.

~ MELODY BEATTIE

give thanks…

Reverence:
leavening every day

In closing, as we began, I am present to the power of gratitude, of living each day with reverence for all of my blessings.

Gratitude is both the first and the final ingredient in my recipe for longevity. Like a leavener in baking, which causes breads to rise and expand, gratitude lifts and evolves our state of mind and body. Regardless of circumstances, when we truly acknowledge our blessings and communicate from our heart, we feel better, softer and more at peace. We blossom and expand. When we are able to be grateful for *all* of our life, every moment, every aspect… life as we know it… is transformed.

Most of us find it fairly easy to be grateful for a beautiful day when everything has gone our way, or we receive a welcome gift or gesture. It is usually more challenging to be inherently grateful for the totality of our lives — to feel and express appreciation for what we commonly refer to as hardships. However, it is precisely these hardships that stretch us the most, bringing about our significant learning, and evolving us into who we are. Usually, the sooner we feel gratitude, the sooner we see light at the end of the tunnel, and our circumstances shift.

We have most commonly been raised to believe that life happens, that things happen to us — "bad things" for no good reason. Sometimes we believe we are "lucky" and there are fortuitous occurrences, and other times we are not so lucky. If we instead choose to embrace and trust *that we are the creators and draw to us what we need*, it is eventually easier to be appreciative for all of life. For when we are creating our life, there is no one else to blame.

What if it is all perfect? What if you are a spirit here in a physical body to learn and evolve? What if we need all of these experiences to teach us what we came here to learn? When this kind of thinking informs our personal philosophy, life is very different, and blame gives way to a humble reverence that enhances every ingredient in our life.

A New Perspective

A few decades ago when I met Michael Shaffer, my chiropractor, and the man that was to become one of my greatest teachers, he asked me a memorable and life-altering question. I was sharing — more aptly complaining about — challenges in my life. I went on for some time, while he sat listening. Michael responded by asking, "Why do you always want things to be easy?"

At first I thought for certain I had heard him incorrectly, then it felt like my jaw fell open. I immediately, and defensively, retorted, "What kind of a question is that? Why wouldn't I want it to be easy? Everyone wants it to be easy." He paused with a soft smile and responded with, "Not me." Needless to say the conversation gave me something to chew on for a while, and I still revisit the flavors to this day. As I reflected on our conversation and on my life, I began to slowly see things anew.

It took a while to truly embrace being grateful for all of the hills and the valleys of my life. I began to see everything and everyone as a teacher and an opportunity for me to grow. If I was short on work, it was an opportunity for me to *be*, rather than to *do*. It was a time for reflection, and to bring balance. I came to see and appreciate the importance of breathing in and breathing out in my life. When my marriage dissolved, I was able to evolve in new ways. The sense of freedom and lightness of being that one acquires from this shift in perspective is extremely rejuvenating! I no longer blame others or circumstances for the events in my life.

When we truly embrace that we are the creators of our life, and are grateful for every aspect, life is less stressful. Less stress, as we know, is a primary ingredient for longevity. When we feel that we have no control of our lives, and live every day with that stress, it can take a toll on our immune system and our well-being.

Even though, in the beginning, it might feel overwhelming to embrace the idea of being in the driver's seat, in time, just like learning a new yoga pose, we can embrace it. We can enjoy being there, the nuances, the newfound strength. We learn patience anew. We come to see our follies in a new light, and hopefully find a sense of humor to help ease the bumps, or occasional hurdles, in the road.

Do not pray for easy lives. Pray to be stronger...
Do not pray for tasks equal to your powers. Pray for powers equal to your tasks.
Then the doing of your work shall be no miracle, but you shall be the miracle.

- PHILLIPS BROOKS
(1835 -1893)

Ways to Practice Reverence

Pythagorus said, "Above all things, reverence thyself." It doesn't matter if your body doesn't yet reflect the ideal health, weight, or beauty that you think it "should." Begin trusting that you are in the perfect place, for this moment, with gratitude for *all* of your life. Every day is a new beginning, and a gift to behold, and "should" is a good word to drop out of your vocabulary!

For me, reverence is a daily appreciation for all of life, for everything contributes to who I am. My days begin by pausing with gratitude for a new day. I feel gratitude throughout the day, and bring closure to my day with appreciation. I love closing my eyes and drawing my hands together in prayer position at my heart.

When we pause, putting our attention on what we have, not what we want or don't have, our energy shifts. Our emotions are lifted, and our stress or concerns do not have the same hold on us.

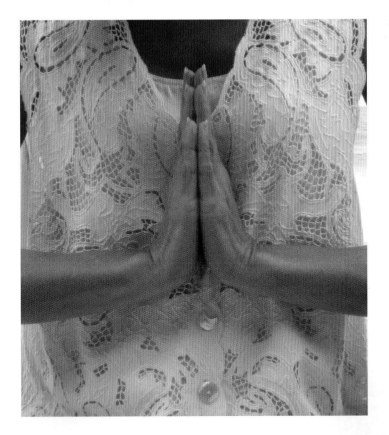

SHARING GRATITUDE

Every day, acknowledge at least three things that you are grateful for that occurred that day. I do this with my family before our evening meal. Our appreciations often lead into insightful stories about our days.

Gratitude journals can also be a richly rewarding experience. Experiment with writing your appreciations about the people, the small things that enlivened a moment, the animals or birds that visited your day or your dreams, the flowers or trees that were blooming, aromas that wafted your way, the sweetness of a ripe piece of fruit, artwork that moved you, sounds that drifted in, or how the sunshine or rain felt upon your body.

May you deepen your discovery as to how infinitely abundant your life is daily, for miracles occur every moment. Appreciate your life and you'll feel more youthful everyday!

BEING OF SERVICE

I find that when we are most challenged is when it is best to step away from our struggles and help another. It's beautiful to experience how, when we stop focusing on our challenges and help someone else, our own issues can shift and lose the hold they had on us. A good exercise in realizing how much you have to be grateful for often begins by going out and helping someone or something that is in greater need.

"It is one of the most beautiful compensations of life, that no man can sincerely try to help another without helping himself."

- *RALPH WALDO EMERSON*

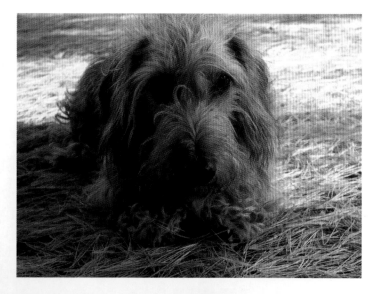

"I think dogs are the most amazing creatures; they give unconditional love. For me they are the role model for being alive."

- *GILDA RADNER*

PAYING HOMAGE TO OUR ANCESTORS

It is valuable to our health and longevity to be grateful for our ancestors who walked before us, not to judge them or hold grudges about what they did or didn't do in their lifetimes. It is not ours to judge another but rather to trust that what they did was perfect, and that their lives contributed in many ways that we will never know, in forming who we are. Affirm, *"I am reverent for what is, what was, and what will be."*

If you look deeply into the palm of your hand, you will see your parents and all generations of your ancestors. All of them are alive in this mo-ment. Each is present in your body. You are the continuation of each of these people.

~ THICH NHAT HANH
VIETNAMESE MONK,
ACTIVIST & WRITER

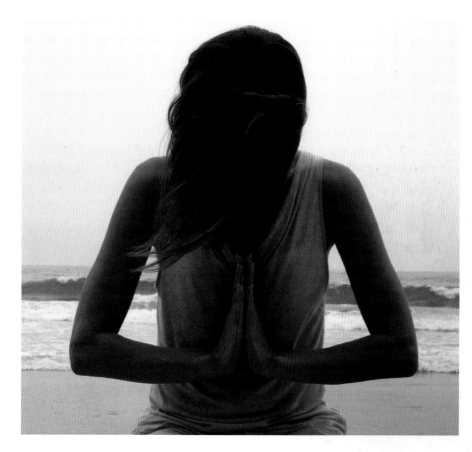

My Thanks To You

Thank you for embracing your well-being and taking conscious steps to make a difference. For everything that you do touches all of life. We are all connected.

May this recipe for longevity help illuminate your path of self-discovery, nourish your evolution, and bring greater peace and fulfillment to your soul. Here's to feeling, thinking and being more youthful — above and beyond what you formerly thought possible — by beginning with simply fifteen minutes of your time throughout your day.

May you live your every day to its fullest with renewed joy, appreciation and delight. To your radiant longevity, to sipping daily from this infinite Fountain of Youth, to connecting all of life and to paying forward the wisdom that we are blessed to receive… cheers!

Namaste.
(the light within me honors and bows to the light within you)

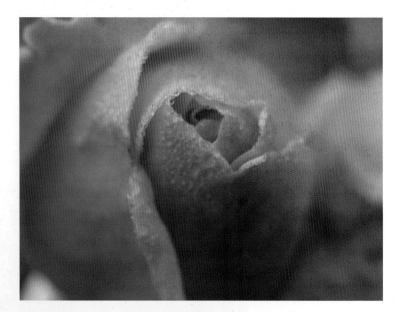

And there came a day when the risk to remain tight in a bud was more painful than the risk it took to blossom.

~ ANAIS NIN

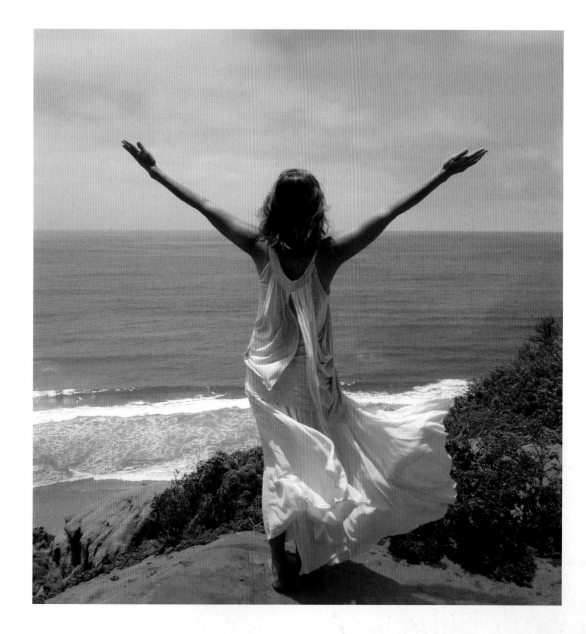

*There is a fountain of youth: it is your mind, your talents,
the creativity you bring to your life and the lives of the people you love.
When you learn to tap this source, you will truly have defeated age.*

~ SOPHIA LOREN

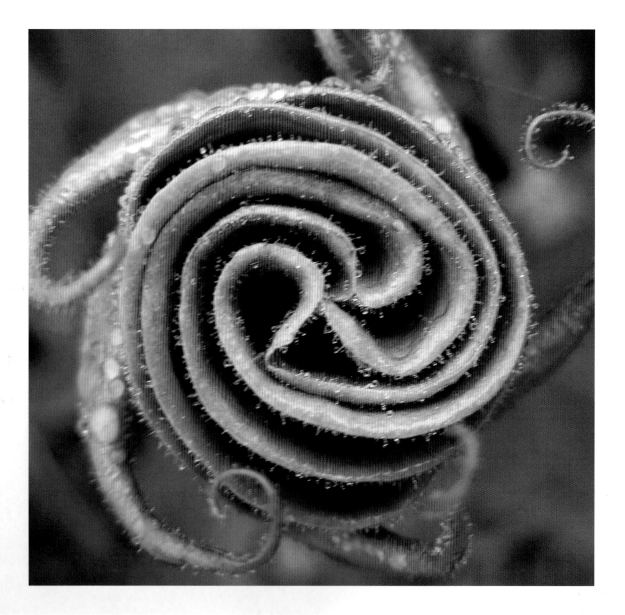

What is right for one soul may not be right for another.
It may mean having to stand on your own and do something strange
in the eyes of others. But do not be daunted,
do whatever it is because you know within it is right for you.

~ EILEEN CADDY

Resources:
for further research on ingredients

The following pages offer more ingredients toward discovering what is best for you, at this moment in your life. Please check my website, *naomicall.com* for a current list. Longevity is an ongoing inquiry and transformation. Here are some favorites.

Make everyday Thanksgiving. Savor, with gratitude, *every flavor of your life*. The bitter, the pungent, the salty, the sour and the sweet.

And now… it's time to create your recipe. Please feel free to share your thoughts and your "recipes" at *naomicall.com*.

Bon Appetit!

And in the end,
it's not the years
in your life that count,
it's the life in your years.

~ *ABRAHAM LINCOLN*

Resources

Books on Healthy Food and Lifestyle

Rainbow Green Live-Food Cuisine, Gabriel Cousens, MD. See also *Conscious Eating, Depression Free for Life*, and *There is a Cure for Diabetes.*

Tree Of Life Rejuvenation Center. Please also see information on Tree Of Life Rejuvenation Center, *www.treeoflife.nu*

Raw for 30. A very inspiring documentary on curing Diabetes.

Eating for Beauty, David Wolfe (one of my favorites), *Superfoods: The Food and Medicine of the Future, The Sunfood Diet Success System and Naked Chocolate: The Astounding Truth about the World's Greatest Food.* His Longevity Now program is a wealth of information. *www.bestdayever.com*

More health-related titles you may wish to consider

The ph Miracle: Balance Your Diet, Reclaim Your Health, Robert O. Young PhD and Shelley Redford Young - This is a great entry level book into healthy eating. I received this book as a gift from a student in her 70s who was ecstatic with it!

Eating Animals, Jonathon Safran Foer

The Calcium Bomb, Douglas Mulhall & Katja Hansen

The China Study, T. Colin Campbell

Earthing, Clinton Ober

Milk - The Deadly Poison, Robert Cohen

Natural Chi Movement, Tienko Ting

… a few Cookbooks

Diet for a New America, John Robbins

Raw Food Made Easy for 1 or 2 People, Jennifer Cornbleet

Becoming Raw - The Essential Guide to Raw Vegan Diets, Brenda Davis, RD and Vesanto Melina, MS, RD.

Nourishing Traditions: The Cookbook that Challenges Politically Correct Nutrition, Sally Falon

Recipes for Life from God's Garden, Rhonda J. Malkmus

Organic food sources

www.sunorganicfarm.com - Nuts, seeds, oil, spices.

www.Mountainroseherbs.com - Fresh, organic herbs and spices.

www.lovestreetlivingfoods.com - Organic foods, supplements, supplies, etc.

www.seaweed.net - Mendocino Sea Vegetable Company.

www.alcasoft.com - Maine Seaweed Company.

www.genefitnutrition.com - Young untreated Thai coconuts.

www.localharvest.org - Lists farmers markets, family farms, and sources for food grown locally in your area.

Inspiration to enlighten and delight your Spirit…

You Can Heal Your Life, Louise Hay. This is an international bestseller. Louise Hay has many inspirational titles that are great books to come back to over and over.

Key To Yourself Opening the Door to A Joyful Life from Within, Venice Bloodworth Ph. D. The book that enlightened me, written in 1952, a shining star.

Taking the Leap: Freeing Ourselves from Old Habits and Fears, Pema Chodron. She has a number of inspiring titles to choose from.

The Art of Happiness, the Dalai Lama. Or you may wish to consider some of his other titles, of which there are many.

Peace is Every Step: The Path of Mindfulness in Everyday Life, Thich Nhat Hahn, Arnold Kotler, and H. H. the Dalai Lama.

The Power of Now, Eckhart Tolle.

Essential Oils & Aromatherapy to soothe and heal

www.youngliving.com - Aromatherapy oils and products.

www.oshadiusa.com - Organic & wildcrafted essential oils & products.

Rebounders… start bouncing your way to great Health!

www.needakusa.com - The best on the market. It's good not to compress on suspension.

Resources

Websites & video clips for healthful information

www.abraham-hicks.com - Inspirational Law of Attraction, positive thinking support.

www.devakant.com - Beautiful music for the soul to accompany your chi, meditation or yoga practices.

www.consciousmedianetwork.com - Highly informative web site.

www.gersontapes.com - The Gerson Tapes, alternative therapies to heal the body.

www.healthfetch.org - A website that features health news feeds from popular websites.

www.johnrobbins.info - Tools, research & information.

www.maritaliving.com - Monthly on-line journal of healthy living tips and insights.

www.mercola.com - Dr. Joseph Mercola's natural health website. Breaking health news and studies.

www.naturalnews.com - Mike Adams natural health site. Over 25, 000 articles on health and healing.

www.notmilk.com - Insightful information on health issues of dairy consumption.

www.rawfoodexplained.com - Website with info on raw food and nutrition theory.

www.rawforlife.com - Information and recipes.

www.renegadehealth.com - The Renegade Health Show, daily short videos on healthy living.

More helpful products and where to find them

DRY BRUSHES

www.naturalhealthtechniques.com - Nice description of how to dry brush the skin and why, and they of course sell dry brushes.

EARTHING PRODUCTS

www.earthinginstitute.net - Provides information for obtaining Earthing products and tips on staying Earthed.

HEALTHY SHOES… NEXT BEST THING TO BARE FEET

www.trueshu.com - Handmade leather moccasins without rubber soles to connect you directly to the Earth for maximum healing benefits.

NETTIE POTS

www.himalayaninstitute.org - Sells nettie pots, a very helpful product and they also offer a host of other products and services.

ORGANIC YOGA STRAPS

www.naomicall.com - organic hemp straps - free of plastic and metal

Informing Yourself About Pesticides

www.beyondpesticides.org

www.foodnew.org

www.foodirradiation.org

www.safelunch.org

www.ewg.org/sites/bodyburden1/ - Environmental Working Group - Excellent site for information on toxics in our lives in our foods, products, homes etc.

Life is all about Water

Water and Salt The Essence of Life, Barbara Hendel & Peter Ferreira.

Tapped Trailer - Explanation of our water situation. *www.youtube.com/watch?v=72MCumz5lq4*

Your Body's Many Cries for Water, Dr. F. Batmanghelidj "You're not sick; you're thirsty. Don't treat thirst with medication." Insightful publication also availble in audio form.

www.findaspring.com - Lists springs in the U.S. and other counties.

Centers & Retreats for Raw & Healthy Living & Yoga Classes

www.gerson.org - The Gerson Institute is a non-profit organization dedicated to providing education and training in the alternative, non-toxic treatment of cancer and other disease.

www.hacres.com - Hallelujah Acres® is a non-denominational ministry that provides education, products, services, and other resources to help people understand and practice God's ways to ultimate health.

Resources

www.hippocratedinst.org - Raw food retreats: treatment for acute and chronic conditions; fasting; raw food preparation training.

www.himalayaninstitute.org - total rejuvenation and education, Pennsylvania.

www.kripalu.org - Kripalu Center for Yoga & Health - for a wide variety of health related classes, workshops and retreats. Yoga certification is also available.

www.optimumhealth.org - Fasting and renewal, education & lifestyle, San Diego, Ca.

www.rawfoodchef.com - Classes, consultation, training, videos, Living Light Culinary Institute.

www.treeoflife.nu - For a totally raw food renewing retreat. Dr. Gabriel Cousens in Patagonia, Arizona.

Alternative Cancer therapies

www.cancerdecisions.com - Healing Cancer from Inside Out by Mike Anderson, DVD and book. Why traditional treatment doesn't work and alternatives you can do.

Cancer, Nutrition, and Healing, Jerry Brunetti, DVD. Told that without chemotherapy he would be dead in six months, he healed his aggressive form of lymphoma using food and supplements. That was more than six years ago.

Knockout: Interviews with Doctors Who Are Curing Cancer and How to Prevent Getting It in the First Place, Suzanne Somers.

Anticancer, David Sevran-Schreiber. He writes about practices that can help prevent and heal cancer, as adjuncts to traditional treatment. Includes resources, such as lists of foods that are healing for specific types of cancer.

Essential dental information

Whole Body Dentistry: Discover the Missing Piece to Better Health, Mark A. Breiner

www.hugginsappliedhealing.com - valuable resources and holistic dentists.

... on fasting, cleansing & juicing

www.ejuva.com - One of the most pure, and conscious colon cleanses available.

www.vitamix.com - the best smoothie maker.

www.thesproutpeople.com - for one of the best greens juicers.

Healing in the Age of Enlightenment, Stanley Burroughs.

Inspirational DVDs for eating healthier cuisine

Food Inc - Excellent documentary on the current state of food.

Food Matters - fabulous interviews and facts about our nutrition and how to use food as medicine.

May I Be Frank? - *mayibefrankmovie.com* - Follows the transformational journey of an overweight man with health concerns as he embraces a raw cuisine.

Raw in 30 days - Inspiring truth about food and curing Diabetes.

Supersize Me - Follows a healthy man through 30 days on a McDonald's diet.

FINDHORN PRESS

Life Changing Books

For a complete catalogue,
please contact:

Findhorn Press Ltd
117-121 High Street,
Forres IV36 1AB,
Scotland, UK

t +44 (0)1309 690582
f +44 (0)131 777 2711
e info@findhornpress.com

or consult our catalogue online
(with secure order facility) on
www.findhornpress.com

For information on the Findhorn Foundation:
www.findhorn.org